DETOX
FOR
WOMEN

Also by Natalia Rose

The Raw Food Detox Diet
Raw Food Life Force Energy

DETOX FOR WOMEN

AN ALL NEW APPROACH FOR
A SLEEK BODY AND RADIANT
HEALTH IN FOUR WEEKS

NATALIA ROSE

WILLIAM MORROW
An Imprint of HarperCollins*Publishers*

This book is written as a source of information only. The information contained in this book should by no means be considered a substitute for the advice of a qualified medical professional, who should always be consulted before beginning any new diet or other health program. The author and the publisher expressly disclaim responsibility for any adverse effects arising from the use or application of the information contained herein.

DETOX FOR WOMEN. Copyright © 2009 by Natalia Rose. All rights reserved. Printed in the United States of America. No part of this book may be used or reproduced in any manner whatsoever without written permission except in the case of brief quotations embodied in critical articles and reviews. For information, address HarperCollins Publishers, 10 East 53rd Street, New York, NY 10022.

HarperCollins books may be purchased for educational, business, or sales promotional use. For information, please write Special Markets Department, HarperCollins Publishers, 10 East 53rd Street, New York, NY 10022.

FIRST EDITION

Designed by Laura Kaeppel

Library of Congress Cataloging-in-Publication Data

Rose, Natalia.
    Detox for Women : an all new approach for a sleek body and radiant health in 4 weeks / Natalia Rose. — 1st ed.
        p. cm.
    Includes index.
    ISBN 978-0-06-174970-4
    1. Detoxification (Health) 2. Women—Health and hygiene. 3. Women—Nutrition. I. Title.

    RA784.5.R67 2009
    613—dc22

                                                            2008047235

09 10 11 12 13   OV/RRD   10 9 8 7 6 5 4 3 2 1

For women everywhere—
may we always seek to lift each other up.

Contents

Foreword

"Let food be thy medicine and medicine be thy food."
—HIPPOCRATES

Having practiced cardiology for the past twenty years, I find it alarming that despite the increased amount of evidence demonstrating the benefits of eating raw and unprocessed food, Americans seem to have lost their nutritional way. They find it very difficult, if not impossible, to change their lifestyle to a healthier one. So I am especially happy to see that in this book, *Detox for Women*, Natalia Rose, an accomplished author and student of nutrition, has tackled the psychological and physical complexities driving America's eating habits. She leads us out of the darkness and into the light of a healthy dietary and low-stress lifestyle synonymous with longer life, free of many chronic diseases.

Most of us in the United States and Western Europe were born of parents who were raised in the 1920s, 1930s, 1940s, and 1950s. These were times, except perhaps for the periods of the Great Depression and during World War II, when food was plentiful and the growth of the meat, dairy, and tobacco industries was meteoric. Nutrition, based on the inclusion of meat, dairy products, vegetables, and grains, and often described as a food pyramid to follow by governmental agencies, was always portrayed as wholesome and nutritionally complete. Many mornings growing up included a "hearty" breakfast of eggs, bacon, sausage, or ham, and fried potatoes, washed down with a glass of whole milk. However, to feed the growing demand for the meat, potato, and dairy staples, industry supported plant and animal science to find ways to enhance crop and feed production using new fertilizers and effective pesticides, to make cattle, chicken, and pork farms more efficient and cost-effective, to increase the milk production of individual cows, and to reduce infectious contamination of products after the animals were sacrificed. The thought never occurred to me as I was entering medical school that food, in our society, was so closely related to some of the most dreaded chronic diseases, such as gastrointestinal disease, rheumatoid arthritis, cardiovascular disease, and cancer.

We have been conditioned to believe that "living and eating well" are birthrights, and we start to follow a lifestyle of excess at an early age. Obesity, a well-defined marker of poor nutrition, was something that happened to poor souls who couldn't control their eating and/or didn't exercise regularly. However, obesity in our society does not affect a minority of citizens, it affects the majority. Obesity in Western society is the direct result of poor nutrition. Poor nutrition (defined as regular consumption of animal meats, dairy products, and processed grains) has been associated epidemiologically with a multitude of chronic diseases affecting the gastrointestinal system, the cardiovascular system, the lungs, the endocrine system, the immune system, the nervous system, the joints, and the skin. Poor nutrition has been directly linked to lethal events such as myocardial infarction, stroke, cancer, respiratory insufficiency, immune deficiency, and accelerated aging. The impact of the addition of tobacco consumption to poor nutrition has long been recognized as a world health problem and continues to grow due to the enabling policies of both government and commercial interests.

Epidemiologic evidence suggests that Western-style diets rich in animal meats, fatty foods, added fats, desserts, and sweets are associated with a substantially increased risk for obesity, type II diabetes, hypertension, and coronary heart disease. Dietary patterns that are characterized by a "healthy" diet high in fruit, vegetables, whole grains, fish, and small amounts of poultry are associated with a lower risk of these diseases. These associations are stronger for dietary patterns than for individual foods, highlighting the importance of identifying and changing foods that are in excess and adding foods that are too limited in the diet. Lifestyle interventions have been shown to have results comparable or superior to drug therapy. As an example, in the *Diabetes Prevention Study*, diet and exercise were more effective than metformin in preventing people with impaired glucose tolerance from progressing to diabetes. In addition to improvements to patient health, lifestyle-oriented change can be cost-effective, especially in high-risk groups.

Over the past fifty years the dietary lifestyle that has undergone the most extensive study has been the so-called Mediterranean diet. The Mediterranean diet is a modern nutritional recommendation inspired by the traditional dietary patterns of some of the countries of the Mediterranean Basin. Based on food patterns typical of Crete, much of the rest of Greece, and southern Italy in the early 1960s, this diet, in addition to regular physical activity, emphasizes abundant plant foods, fresh fruit as the typical daily dessert, olive oil as the principal source of fat, minimal dairy products (principally cheese and yogurt), fish and poultry consumed in low to moderate amounts, zero to four eggs consumed weekly, high levels of dietary fiber, red meat consumed in very low amounts, and wine consumed in low to moderate amounts. Total fat in this diet is 25 percent to 35 percent of total calories, with saturated fat at 8 percent or less of total calories.

These reported benefits of the Mediterranean diet represent an apparent paradox: although the people living in Mediterranean countries tend to consume relatively high amounts of fat, they have far lower rates of cardiovascular disease than countries like the United States, where similar levels of total fat consumption are found. One of the obvious differences is the large amount of "healthy fat" (olive oil, avocado, etc.) used in the Mediterranean diet. The other main differences include the greater proportion of green vegetables, fruits, legumes, and unprocessed grains compared to the average American diet. Unlike the high amount of animal and dairy fats typical to the American diet that raise cholesterol, healthy fats lower cholesterol levels in the blood. The diet also is known to lower blood sugar levels and blood pressure, and recently was demonstrated to prevent the development of diabetes in a large series. A nearly 50 percent reduction in the risk of developing chronic obstructive lung disease and emphysema has also been demonstrated in patients on this diet.

What is important to emphasize is that the preference for fresh fruit and vegetables in the Mediterranean diet will result in a higher consumption of raw foods, a lower production and ingestion of cooking-related oxidants, and a consequent decreased waste of nutritional and endogenous antioxidants. The high intake of antioxidants and fiber helps to scavenge even the small amount of oxidants or oxidized compounds. Removal of oxidants from the body has been shown to reduce the oxidation of low-density lipoproteins (LDL), important in retarding the formation of atherosclerotic plaque.

It is also now understood that the explanation of the benefit of this lifestyle is not any particular nutrient or supplement, but the *combination* of nutrients found in raw and unprocessed food. This is the gold nugget that tends to get buried in reports that the Mediterranean diet will make you young by letting you drink wine. And this is also where *Detox for Women* is a standout in the field of nutritional literature. Natalia Rose carefully analyzes the reasons for our current predicament, with thoughtful references to her own real struggles, and shows women step-by-step how to transition from unhealthy to healthy. Through her unique approach of eating healthy, predominately raw foods and regularly cleansing (de-toxifying) the intestinal tract of putrefied matter and unhealthy microorganisms and yeast, the reader is taken to new levels of health with enhanced organ system function and mental clarity that far exceed what is achieved on the Mediterranean diet.

Detox for Women also highlights the hormonal differences in the female body and the overwhelmingly acidic environment that facilitate the physical and emotional changes most women experience living and eating in the western hemisphere. Natalia shows readers why they experience such dramatic results and shows them how to find a way to better health. This book should be mandatory reading for all women who care about themselves and their families, especially for teenage girls, who have the opportunity at their young age to dramatically affect their life and longevity by adopting the healthiest of lifestyles.

JOHN E. STROBECK, MD, PHD

Introduction

Detox: Is It Extremely Radical or Extremely Rational?

Sometimes we have to make a radical choice to bring ourselves back into balance. Sometimes, the thing that seems the most off-the-wall is actually the most sane and rational choice. In our case, as women circa 2009, we have lived in such extreme conditions dietetically and environmentally that the only way to restore our bodies, minds, and spirits to wholeness is to take a giant leap in the opposite direction—back toward truth.

While it does not seem extreme to the modern woman to live and eat per the social norms of the day, the body was not actually designed for donuts, bagels and cream cheese, lattes, chicken wraps, vodka tonics, diet sodas, and air-conditioned office jobs. The modern woman, however, is very much conditioned to these things, and to consider living another way can be *very* scary. I totally understand; in fact . . .

. . . when I first heard of someone following a cleansing/detox diet fifteen years ago, I thought, "Wow, I could never do that. It sounds so extreme. They sure must have a lot of willpower." But, lo and behold, for the last ten years I have been practicing and, yes, *enjoying* a cleansing diet-lifestyle!

When the time is right, people can do things that they would otherwise have thought impossible. There was a time when I could not even imagine giving up sugar. I remember it clearly. My esthetician was following a strict Candida cleanse and the mere thought of not being able to eat my beloved frozen yogurt (strictly verboten on "the cleanse") sounded unfathomable to me at the time. If I had listened to her back then I probably wouldn't have needed the facials for my copious breakouts that she was there to extract!

Back then I was just as addicted to these foods as you may be today. I couldn't imagine not eating frozen yogurt, bread, muffins, steak, etc. But as I gradually became more and more unwell and desperate both physically and emotionally for a better life, "detox fare" started to look more and more appealing. My choice was quite simple: either I would stay sick and heavy and deteriorate more over time, or I would accept the fact that I was living out of harmony with natural law and correct it.

I should add that I was also a serious "foodie"—taste and hearty quantities ruled my world. The thing is, I still want my meals to be delicious and hearty. The difference is I now know how to have it all: I simply got creative and adapted what I knew about how to make food delicious (which I will share with you) to what I know about what works best in the female body. I get the best of both worlds! In fact, I cannot remember the last time I was eating out with friends when they didn't specifically mention that they wished they had ordered what I was eating. Some even ask me to order for them outright. This way, they know they'll get something delicious that will leave them feeling amazing without a "food hangover" later.

People do not have to have the rug pulled out from under them to detox. But there are restrictions. If you can just hang in there long enough to see the payoff you will no longer perceive that which you give up as being such a sacrifice. Ultimately, if the food you get to eat tastes really flavorful, fresh, and hearty, *and* you get to feel and look better than you ever imagined, you're not going to be swayed back to old habits. You'll see, the payoff is huge!

Also, as you clean your system, you'll bring your taste buds back to a normal, balanced state; the need for excessively salty, fatty, starchy foods comes in part from a dulling of the taste buds that takes place over years of eating processed foods. In a short time of eating more simply, your palate will be highly satisfied—even titillated—by naturally flavored foods.

What I'll help you do is strike the perfect balance between food satisfaction and effective physical renewal so that you love the food and love your transformation! There's nothing better than living in a cleansed body. It's pure euphoria.

Because the foods we are going to be emphasizing are not dense, inflammatory, or disturbing to the body in any way, you can enjoy very hearty quantities. Further, remember that the extremes to which we have been eating have caused us to approach food in a really perverse way. We were never meant to eat what is commonly considered "food," particularly in the quantities and as often as we do. We have created social customs and addictions that have thwarted the truth about food. Remember this as you go as it will help when you are in situations where you may be self-conscious of making choices that are so different to what may be practiced around you. While it may feel like you are the one being extreme, it's really the common ways of eating that are extreme—people are just too addicted and invested in their lifestyles to see it.

The Silver Bullet Solution

This book was created to present the silver bullet solution that can get every woman into her best possible state of body and mind. You might be thinking, "That's impossible; each woman is so different—each comes with a different body type, lineage, health history, personality, tastes, etc." Yes, each woman's body is unique. Each woman's reaction to certain foods will differ in some way. Each woman has her own set of food "rules" and fears, yet given all of this, this particular approach is a surefire plan for every woman, as you will soon see!

Every woman from the raw food enthusiast to the long-term health seeker, chronic dieter and mainstream "average" eater (and everything in between) will be served here.

If you're impatient to get started, you can jump to Day 1 of the 30-day "Detox for Women Program" on page 74. However, if you choose to do this, I implore you to read everything leading up to the actual program as soon as you are able so that you fully understand *why* you are doing *what* you are doing.

The commonly accepted diet, health, and exercise notions that have permeated the market over the last thirty years have left the health world in shambles. Vegan women think they have the answers, gym devotees are married to their programs, raw foodists think they have found the "holy grail," and the women that count calories, carbs, and fat grams hold fast to those principles. Meanwhile, most of these dogmatic rules are mixed up with a lot of misunderstandings, as well as sales and marketing agendas, and should be discarded accordingly. It's best to leave behind any diet dogma you have learned. Clinging to old ways of thinking about food will not help you.

While I myself eat a highly raw-vegan diet (with exception of raw goat cheese), I understand the value of non-raw, non-vegan foods. I have direct experience with the benefits and shortcomings of limited dietetic approaches and the great value in transition and flexibility around dietary principles. If you are a vegan and you're doing well as a vegan, you are encouraged to stick to vegan foods as you apply the guidelines. However, cooked foods and animal foods are also included in the broad scope of this program to make it accessible to every woman.

The purpose of this book is to give you your "ace in the hole." Once you know what your best really feels and looks like and you know how to achieve it, you can do as you please (either stick closely to it as most of my female clients do, or weave in and out using it as your lifestyle home base). If you wind up eating other foods or temporarily going back to old lifestyle choices and fall out of that high space, you'll know what to do to get back. Together we'll find diet nirvana. You can decide, after feeling what that's like, if you want to stay there and how to get there whenever you wish.

Here are a few basic guidelines before you proceed, to ensure best results:

- Read the book in its entirety

- Take the test on page 56 to determine which program to start with

- Shop for the basics on the shopping list as needed (page 63)

- Read the introduction to the recipe section to learn how to make natural foods incredibly tasty—there are important *tricks* here that can make the whole program work if you know them, girls!

- Incorporate the dietary plan into your life

- Watch your body transform until you feel you have achieved all your goals

- Return to the book for further guidance and additional levels of integrating the principles as necessary or desired

- Tailor your diet to include any other relatively acceptable foods you enjoy and your body seems to tolerate well

- Pay attention to the nonphysical changes that benefit your social, emotional, and family experiences as detoxification effects healing in all areas of your life!

part one

DETOX FOR WOMEN

Why Detox?

Detoxification is quite possibly the single most important thing we can do to improve our life. When done correctly, it removes all that stands in our way of pure energy, joy, and ideal physical experience. When we share space in our body with substances that do not belong there (created by an unfit diet-lifestyle), we give away our clarity, authenticity, and inner power. When we "de-toxify" (meaning we remove these harmful substances), we find ourselves in unfettered wholeness and thrive.

In my experience, the results of the *Detox for Women* method are powerful and immediate and they last. In fact, health and physique consistently improve over the long term. Here are some of the common reports I receive from my clients who follow this method:

- Rapid, lasting weight loss
- Elimination or marked decrease of cellulite
- Firming and tightening of the facial skin
- Firming and tightening of other areas on the body
- Increased circulation contributing to a healthy glow
- Marked increase in energy throughout the day
- Feelings of natural euphoria
- Improvement of sleeping patterns
- Reduction of wrinkles and under-eye circles
- Decrease in mood swings
- More comfortable menstrual cycles

The Problem Behind the Problem

The root cause of physical, emotional, and mental imbalances is the clogging of our cells, tissues, organs, and pathways due to the residue left behind in the body after decades of an unfit diet-lifestyle. While there are myriad different names for modern diseases in medical literature, there is really just one core cause of all these imbalances: clogging of the cells and pathways due to the accumulation of inappropriate matter left behind. There is also one solution: the removal of that matter. This is the true meaning of detoxification.

When substances are consumed that are not easily digested and passed by the human body, they leave residue behind. This residue starts out in the intestines where it ferments and putrefies and eventually (since the body is an interconnected organism) permeates the tissues of the intestine and circulates throughout the body—winding up in the blood and tissues.

Once the cells are contaminated by this old matter, the healthy microbes in the cells develop into unhealthy, antagonistic bacteria and yeast. As the body accumulates more of this residue, the undesirable strains of bacteria and yeasts proliferate, overthrowing the healthy balance the body needs to fight them off and stay well. The degree to which we experience symptoms or illnesses is directly related to the degree to which our body's tissues have been overcome by bacteria and yeast.

Fight the Good Bacteria Fight

As long as our good bacteria successfully fend off undesirable amounts of unfriendly bacteria, our cells will stay clean and we will not have symptoms or illnesses. If we do have troublesome symptoms and identifiable illnesses, you can be sure it is because these key systems have been compromised through the clogging of the cells and pathways, obstructing the organization of the system and enabling undesirable bacteria and yeast to take hold.

Since waste matter along with sugars and starches from common foods feed the bacteria and yeast, we find ourselves craving more sugars and starches without actually knowing why we are driven to consume them. This is a form of addiction.

You are probably aware that viruses can enter the body from the outside, but in 1883, a scientist by the name of Antoine Beauchamp revealed that viruses are also developed from within. "The primary cause of disease," he discovered, "is in us, always in us." The likelihood of bacteria snowballing into pathogenic viruses or the body becoming infected by pathogenic germs, Beauchamp pointed out, is directly related to the degree to which the body serves as a good host to them (if the body supports their existence). What Beauchamp is saying is that cells that have become defiled with fermentation form pathogens from the inside out!

Once bacteria invade the cells and tissues, we start to show signs of deterioration. The only way to turn the condition around is to stop supporting the proliferation of the rogue bacteria and yeast by removing the waste that supports them. This removal of waste is literally *de-tox-ification*—the removal of the toxins.

Why Detox for Women?

Adult women long for the kind of beauty, physique, and lasting youth that can only be experienced by a clean-celled body. However, the modern woman has a system that has been seriously compromised by lifestyle. These compromises have thrown her healthy microbial balance so completely out of whack that a very specific prescription for detox is necessary. You will find this plan altogether different from others that have been popularized by the raw food and detox movement, and uniquely formulated to produce results in adult women.

While men also suffer from yeast, fungus, and bacteria overgrowth, estrogen, the dominant female hormone, helps to breed yeast for several reasons. An estrogenic environment supports the production of lycogen (the storage form of glucose in animal cells), which is a major food supplier for yeast. Estrogen is also responsible for many of our moods, making women gravitate toward comfort foods—starchy, sugary, and often highly processed, setting the stage for yeast to thrive.

In addition to being more prone to yeast, women also tend to be more acutely sensitized to the symptoms that go along with yeast and bacteria imbalances: bloat, moodiness, poor skin quality, excess weight, etc. We not only feel terrible, we are depressed because we feel the pressure to look perfect all the time. Then to top it off, women quadruple-task their lives away!

Real Woman: Sarah Appleton, Fashion Model, NYC

"I work as a model. I deal with the scrutiny of every inch of my naked body. I have to wear a kind of mask to look glamorous, perfect, and slender at all times. It's really a deception. But I was sucked in by the pressures of the fashion industry and today's society. I spent copious amounts of money and time on every route to be thinner—to have perfect skin and to have what I thought would give me fulfillment. In the end, it was a self-destructive path. I had episodes of mononucleosis, Lyme disease, drug abuse, and depression. I became addicted to shopping. I experienced self-abandonment and self-hatred; I became obsessed with food—overeating, cleansing, fasting, and overexercising. I went through periods of anorexia and bulimia. At one point I was instructed by a gastrointestinal doctor to take laxatives as a solution for a lifelong suffering from IBS and severe constipation, which I turned into a terrifying addiction to laxatives! All this to keep an "acceptable" shell, which was crumbling from the inside out.

"I was lost from myself, relationships, the world, my body, and spiritual being. I have wanted children my whole life. This was becoming seemingly impossible in years to come when my body began to collapse, having just a handful of periods in four years. I had to stop to live a life and have a chance for a family.

"I thank God and the universe for finding Natalia. Her guidance saved my life on levels unimaginable. I am reconnecting my whole being physically, mentally, and spiritually. Empowered by my Life Force Energy that flows through my body as it heals and functions organically, with a special blessing the day my period came back.

"I enjoy amazing juices, veggies, fruits, and foods that make my taste buds explode! My favorites are green lemonade, raw goat cheese, avocados; and I could go on and on. My energy has skyrocketed. I am light, not weighed down by toxic waste. I don't crave foods I used to, and when I step back and think about how great I feel now, I wonder how much I really enjoyed them.

"I care for myself with an assortment of Natalia's simple tools to balance and calm my body. My bath-time calming is a daily gift releasing the day's baggage centering myself. Meditation guides me to a peaceful existence and continues to open my eyes wider and wider. Massage, body brushing, infrared sauna, and colonics with Gil Jacobs are a constant to aid in removing built-up damage and toxicity! Yoga balances me in the world. I now run for pleasure and enjoy Pilates, ballet, and swing class because I think of them as ways to maximize my Life Force Energy, instead of just burning calories, which always felt like torture. My creativity is blossoming again. The simple morning sun is an instant energizer, WOW!

"My physical body has shed the baggage and transformed. I finally have beautiful, glowing, smooth skin. I am present in my life. I am self-confident and feel special to be me. This is a precious feeling I wish upon everyone!"

So you can understand that dietary guidance is useless if it cannot be woven into a woman's home life, social life, and work life and mesh with her spirit and personality. Our physical body is so deeply interconnected with our emotional, mental, and spiritual aspects, food is only part of a full spectrum of support we need to be successful with detoxification. To be truly transformative, all aspects of a woman's inner and outer life must be taken into account. Therefore, a detox program specific to women's needs is absolutely essential.

Something Dire Is Afoot

It dawned on me a couple of years ago that all of a sudden the majority of the women who were coming to see me had all the markings of an overyeasted system; whereas before it was only a handful. This made it impossible for me to recommend classic raw and detox items like fresh fruit, sprouted grain breads, and sweeteners like agave or raw honey. It forced me to structure an approach for these women that was still grounded in my core principles, but also incorporated the measures necessary to fight yeast and bacteria. I was pleased to be able to present them with a powerfully effective program that was also remarkably satisfying to the palate and in some ways even easier to integrate into the modern, busy lifestyle than the original program.

I was still concerned, however, with what was happening with women's systems. This was becoming an overnight epidemic. There was no question that something had changed, making it necessary to offer this modified program to a large percentage of my female clientele. "What was going on and why now?" This was the obvious question I posed to myself.

The answer is that our world is exponentially more acidic and the quality of our food, water, and air is more offensive than it was even just a few years ago. Yeast and bacteria thrive in an acidic environment. When a compromised system is placed in a hostile environment, the system is entirely helpless to defend itself as it otherwise would. The environment had never before been quite so harmful; the organism had never been quite so weakened. I'd also never seen such a stampede of women in need of help. They were coming in droves all with slightly different ailments, but all coming from the same losing battlefield.

Women's health imbalances were serious enough before, but today the balance has been so corrupted that the internal terrain and prognosis for the future has become downright dire.

This problem doesn't have to be scary; it just needs to be addressed clearly and corrected before it is beyond our ability to fix. That would actually be scary.

Detox for Women could not come a moment too soon. We are living in a world where it's no longer an option, but a necessity, for women to cleanse their bodies if they wish to be healthy and live well.

"Curb Appeal" or Real Appeal?

What spirit is so empty and blind, that it cannot recognize the fact that the foot is more noble than the shoe, and skin more beautiful than the garment with which it is clothed?

—MICHELANGELO

Mirror, Mirror on the Cellular Wall . . .

Your face is a magic mirror. In the very texture, color, and terrain you can see into the state of your cells, pathways, and organs. Under-eye circles and puffiness around the eye area reveal the stagnant flow of a body whose essential fluids cannot move rapidly through the system as they were designed to. Loose, wrinkled skin bespeaks of organ tissue that is starved of life force and nutrients. You don't need a fancy medical device to scope out your internal workings. You can just look at your fancy magic mirror. If you're very young you may not see the effects of your poor eating on your face yet because the poisoning has not gone on long enough to permeate your tissues. But if you've been eating "normally" that's just a matter of time.

As you may remember from basic human biology, cells combine to make tissues, which combine to form organs that collectively make up the human organism. The cells are the foundation of our body; all our ills (and wellness) can be traced to the intercellular cleanliness of these infinitesimally small organisms. Healthy and clean human cells conduct an electromagnetic current that I call Life Force Energy. Clean cells act as superconductors of this life current, resulting in a body that glows!

The eyes on a clean-celled woman are naturally bright and her mind is naturally clear (and brilliant, of course). Her skin is naturally toned, taut, and cellulite free. By the same token, the greater accumulation of waste in the body, the less Life Force Energy the cells conduct, and the more rapidly you'll appear to age and deteriorate.

The very simple but profound truth about beauty is: *when the body's cells are clean and the pathways open and flowing, the female body naturally looks lovely and perfect.* Seriously, that's all there is to it. The secret is out! When the body gets clean on the inside a remarkable hidden beauty surfaces—that's what you're going to start to see in the coming weeks!

Do You Want "Curb Appeal" or Real Appeal?

Living out of harmony with the body per the modern diet-lifestyle is what makes the quest for beauty so elusive and laborious for women today. Our modern ways of living diminish a woman's innate beauty potential. If we just make a few intelligent adjustments to our lives, we'll immediately start to reharmonize and awaken our highest beauty potential.

The common approach to caring for the female body, followed by millions of women, actually hastens her deterioration (yes, you read that right). Women have been primping, polishing, and blow-drying, making up their lips and lashes, dieting, squishing their breasts into miracle bras and their feet into pumps, all in the name of beauty and presentation.

I call this approach drugstore beauty; it merely masks the face and body. It just covers up sickness and deterioration. It ignores the truth about the body—how it is made and how it should be maintained. Makeup, volumizing shampoos, whitening toothpastes, nail polish, self-tanners, cellulite creams, antiaging creams, and so on only *cover* a woman's face and body—they create a façade that washes away to reveal the unattractive truth with a little soap and water.

It's a vicious cycle: the modern lifestyle stamps out a woman's youth and beauty with the wrong foods and lifestyles; and then sends her out to buy chemically laden products or drugs to help her try to look younger, more beautiful, and appear healthy! These same products cause further deterioration (many cosmetic items women routinely use daily are loaded with toxins: antiperspirants, tampons, chemically based face and body products, to name a few) and seep poisons in her body that land in her tissues contributing to their damage.

These products only serve to create curb appeal—like a house that looks great from the road, but when you get inside you discover a weak structure and lots of deterioration. The façade is where the appeal ends.

You can bleach your teeth, take medication to bring about clear skin, use concealer to cover darkness under the eyes, enhance your breasts with the right bras, and don pumps that make your legs look longer and slimmer; but underneath it all is a degenerating body whose only hope to keep up appearances is to go further into this false beauty paradigm with every decade attempting to fend off the inner deterioration and preserve the curb appeal. Seeking beauty in the old way has got to stop. It simply doesn't offer any real, lasting radiance.

I'm not saying that we should never use cosmetics or dress creatively. Make-up, hair styles, and wardrobe all have their place in a woman's presentation and are part of the fun and natural inclination women have to be beautiful and creative; but what's happened is that women have focused too much on their outer appearance and overlooked that which actually has the greatest bearing on their appearance, vitality, and state of being, namely: the inner care and upkeep deep in the cells and tissues of their bodies.

Clean cells and open flowing pathways in the body are the only way to ensure true lasting health and beauty. That essential truth lies at the core of any truly effective health and beauty regimen. When we care for the well-being of our cells and inner pathways to ensure that all is flowing well and clean inside, we build a real foundation of beauty, fight aging, and a develop a lovely physique. Yet rarely in all the health and fashion magazines, or in the knowledge handed from grandmother to granddaughter, sister to sister, friend to friend, is there any mention of cellular cleanliness. Instead, ours is a culture that embraces an unfit diet-lifestyle and then attempts to remedy all the physical, emotional, and physiological imbalances that result by applying more inharmonious substances. Sisters, this is madness!

You could be glorious! You could be naturally radiant, naturally thin, naturally joyful, naturally youthful-looking.

FROM CELLULITE TO CELLS YOU LIKE!

As most women know, addressing cellulite with creams and thermal spa treatments is useless. However, women are not doomed to be stuck with their unsightly cellulite. This program helps the body eliminate waste matter, which combines with fluids in the body, making that cottage cheese–like indentation on the skin. The women who do this program report complete or nearly complete elimination of cellulite in just a few months. If they stick with the principles of maintenance, it will not reappear.

A Path to Freedom

It's time to develop a new self-care philosophy for women. We need to do this to protect ourselves, our children, and the generations to come. We need to remove the suffering that causes this vicious cycle so women can be free in their bodies and free from anything that would hold them back.

Cleaning the body completely changes one's life experience; it's like the difference between going through life carrying a lead pack and cruising through with wings on our heels. The one holds us down; the other uplifts and propels us forward!

Women are very good at persevering on sheer willpower—pretending they're okay and presenting a face to the world that falsely bespeaks contentment. But when you're weighed down by your body or your inner pain, no matter how good an actress you are, you are suffering and missing out on the pleasures of a free, happy life.

When women are *pretending* that everything is okay, they are not communicating honestly with themselves or each other. The result is that each of us has a terrible sense of isolation, thinking we are the only ones suffering—and that there must be something wrong with us. We wonder why it is so hard for us to measure up to other women who seem so perfect!

I see these women in my office every day and it is just heartbreaking to know how alone they have felt until that moment. Their relief is indescribable, and their healing rapid—once they get the facts straight and learn what's really going on. When an entire generation of women winds up experiencing the same symptoms, that's nature making a great big announcement that something is very much out of harmony with the natural plan.

Let's blow the top off of this charade that breeds more pain, unhealthy competition, and suffering so that real contentment, real joy, and real wellness can supplant this falseness, shall we?

Your True Potential

One thing I have my student teachers practice when they train with me is a game I like to play alone when I walk down the busy streets of New York City. As the masses of people fly by me with their drooping skin, dark circles under their puffy eyes, gas pressure pushing the skeletal structure out of natural alignment, wobbly bits in all sorts of random places, and a general look of dissatisfaction on their faces, I envision them in their perfectly cleansed state—as if the accumulation of their diet and lifestyle had never touched them, or pulled them into the dark world of toxicity, which morphs the body into shapes and the skin into hues unnatural to the design of the perfected human being.

I see them glowing and radiant—what they would be if the nachos, pizza, burgers, soy chips, cow milk, years in the office, oppression of societal norms, and hours in front of computer and television screens never happened. I see their "parallel reality self" that lived in the fresh air and sunlight on mangoes, papayas, and young coconuts in families and communities that held each other in love and joy.

I see their true potential. And I will tell you something; if they could see what I see they would turn it all around and desire it more than money, a new car, the right house, the right social group, the right job, or anything else. If they knew they could feel that way every day they wouldn't trade it for anything.

The human potential is little understood. You have no idea how amazing you can look and feel when gas pressure, waste residue, and all the side effects of improper living leave your cells and tissues! Your individual potential for beauty, health, and general love for life is much greater than you think it is.

Dissatisfaction with life, a dull appearance, dry hair, brittle nails, "cottage cheese" thighs, loose skin, chubby ankles and chin—these are not you. These are just you on the modern lifestyle. I've seen women morph from pudgy, bloated, rapidly aging, depressed heavyweights into completely new beings. You can stop dwelling on the minutiae of your perceived flaws and nagging imperfections now because those little things will all go away when your body is cared for correctly and cleansed!

Pop Yourself the Question

So here we are at a moment of new revelation on the body's ills and proper diet. The call: To turn our backs on the social norms and our internal programming and allow truth to guide our choices instead.

In my experience, it's important to make a formal acknowledgement of your decision to move in a new direction, and draw a line in the sand between former ways of living and thinking and a more advanced ideal. It forces one to see the higher good and then set out to follow it. You can only do your best, but if you follow the highest you know and you are confident about why you are doing it, chances are you will elevate your diet and your life experience rather quickly.

So here is your opportunity for the "moment of truth." Stake your claim to the balanced, beautiful, female body and make that choice!

Okay, it's official—you're on board. You're committed. Let's discover how to care for the female body:

Time for Detox!

Real Woman: Susie Castillo, Actress, Los Angeles, CA

Susie is an actress, the author of *Confidence Is Queen*, and a former Miss America (2003) and Miss Teen USA. She came in to see me with her husband, Matt. She epitomizes what I call "The New Beauty"—a beauty that reflects real health, joy, and spirit within. This program was created with her very much in mind.

"I'm both fortunate and unfortunate in that I've always been pretty slim, regardless of my diet. If that doesn't make sense, let me explain. From the outside I looked healthy. I was slim and active, so I assumed I was healthy on the inside as well. But that's exactly what was unfortunate about it. . . . I wasn't.

"I was raised by a strict, old-school Puerto Rican mother and grandmother. At every meal, if I left any food on my plate, they would remind me that there were starving children in Africa who wish they had food to eat. It made me feel terrible, so I would eat everything!

"To make matters worse, I wasn't eating healthy foods. My mom's cooking typically consisted of white rice, beans, fried chicken, and fried sweet plantains for dinner . . . yikes, right!? But it tasted OHHH so good. Then as I got into my mid-twenties, that Puerto Rican food was starting to lead to some Puerto Rican curves.

"For a young woman working in the entertainment industry, curves are not what you'd call "acceptable." The more you weigh the more you reduce the odds of getting or retaining a job. It's sad but true. Most actors and hosts were thin and I began to feel the pressure to lose weight. It had been my dream since I was a little girl to be on TV and there I was living in New York City, working as a host for MTV . . . I wasn't gonna blow it! My publicist had just informed me that *Maxim* magazine wanted to feature me in an upcoming issue and I had two months to prepare for the photo shoot . . . OMG!

"But I wanted to get into shape in a healthy way. So, I began to dig for information about nutrition. I'd read fitness magazines, watch the news, and monitor diet trends which led to me eating all organic foods while avoiding fried and processed foods. I would also work out longer and harder, all while cutting back on food portions because I always thought I ate too much (no exaggeration, I can eat just as much food as my 6'1", 210 lb. husband!). I thought that going to the gym 5-6 times per week and cutting my portions would be the answer. However, what quickly followed were feelings of guilt any time I ate too much or had my favorite soufflé at Morton's Steakhouse. And when I controlled my portions, I was left unsatisfied . . . and still hungry! I hated it and I found myself miserable about eating!

"Still, I thought I was doing pretty well. But what I wasn't doing was getting to the heart of the matter. My husband, Matt, and I were reading mainstream media that said what we should eat and not eat, but we weren't learning anything about how the human body really works.

"Then we met Natalia Rose. I believe the story of how I found Natalia was one of destiny. One day at a fabulous Manhattan event, I just happened to meet a friend of hers: fitness trainer Alastair Greer. I was looking for a nutritionist, so I asked him if he knew of any good ones that he could recommend. The first and only name he mentioned, and emphatically, was Natalia Rose.

"To make a long story short, as of this writing, Matt and I have been properly combining and juicing for about a year and a half and we absolutely love it. We never got sick and actually can't remember the last time we were!

"I'm so grateful to have found Natalia and her priceless knowledge. I have been enlightened and the quality of life for my family and myself has improved dramatically because we are so much healthier. The best part is that I don't EVER want to stray from the diet because I know what is going to happen inside if I do. Diet trends have never explained to me why I'm eating a certain way. They say "eat this and you'll be thin and healthy" . . . that's it. There's no education. Because of Natalia I now have an understanding of how food behaves in our digestive system and how our bodies function. I know the purpose of it all and that knowledge is definitely empowering!"

part two

THREE STEPS TO DETOX

Step #1: Starve the Yeast

The first step in cleansing the body is to take every possible measure to prevent offering yeast and bacteria anything to dine on! There are several unavoidable laws of nature that we will discuss in this book—the one most essential to understanding how to prevent harmful yeast and bacteria overgrowth is the following: An environment of waste from food left between 40° and 100° Fahrenheit will ferment and putrefy, thus breeding yeast and bacteria. All the calorie and carb counting in the world can't help you if your cells are festering with this stuff.

The appearance of acne, eczema, and psoriasis emerging from the skin is a perfect example of bacteria and yeast infesting human tissue (in this case, the skin). Off-putting though it may be, we need to see how these skin conditions actually reveal what is occurring inside the body. But if we know where physical problems originate we can solve them. Covering up skin eruptions with medication just diffuses the sound of the body's alarm bell; piling cosmetics over them, likewise, will never remedy the root cause. The symptoms will keep reappearing and ultimately ransack our organs as the waste is pushed deeper into the tissue because of the prolonged suppression.

One main reasons I believe teens suffer from such dire skin eruptions (pimples, acne) is that after twelve or thirteen years of an unfit diet, the tissue poisoning has reached a critical mass; it now is showing up on the exposed tissue (the skin). Changing hormones and oily skin will certainly exacerbate this condition, but teenage breakouts were not common prior to industrialization. The unfit lifestyle can negatively impact the balance of hormone secretions coming from the endocrine system; but that is a symptom of imbalance, not the cause.

MEDICATIONS AND YEAST

In addition to the overwhelming intake of flour and sugar in the Western diet, the other major contributing factor to yeast in women is medication, predominantly antibiotics and hormones like those found in HRT and birth control pills. Progesterone feeds *Candida albicans* and estrogen supports glycogen, which yeast feeds on. If you have a history of taking these medications, birth control or HRT, or antibiotics, the likelihood of a yeast overgrowth and the symptoms that go with it is high and must be treated accordingly before you can ever hope to lose weight or feel good. Even if you have a history of eating meats, chicken, and dairy (other than those raised free to roam by an extremely reputable organic source), you have been unknowingly taking antibiotics by eating the flesh and drinking the milk from hormone- and antibiotic-injected, starch-fed animals. This kills off the susceptible bacteria while it increases the resistant bacteria.

In the same way, bacterial infections in the bronchial tubes, sinuses, bladder, and ears are all evidence of the bacteria from food waste permeating the tissues and contaminating the blood stream. These bacteria are breeding from the inside out. Antibiotics will destroy them temporarily but antibiotics will also kill off their beneficial counterparts. In other words, antibiotics can actually make the imbalance even worse. The only true remedy is to begin steps to detoxify our systems.

The modern way of raising, feeding, killing, and packaging meat renders all arguments for eating meat null and void. A giant "condemned" sign should be plastered industry-wide on these contaminated meats. The entire practice is vile and inhumane. The question now is whether consumers are going to stop behaving like the herd animals they have been conditioned to eat, and bring an end to this practice.

Make no mistake: What you find in the grocery today is "not your daddy's steak."

Detox for Women is a way of living and eating that is superior to any other approach because without the cleaning and maintenance of cells, our body falls apart. All other diets are ineffective because nothing else takes into consideration the essential foundation of the environment for human tissues. With the exception of a strict anti-candida diet (which has its own shortcomings) every other approach either feeds bacteria and yeast, or constipates. This breeds and feeds more bacteria through the accumulation of acid waste by-products (such as in the case of the high-protein diets).

There is a way to turn this all around and wind up on the right side of natural law without being uncomfortably strict. Returning the body to balance and inner cleanliness doesn't require an ultra-strict diet. We don't need to completely "red light" sugars and starches to correct a moderate yeast imbalance; we just need to "yellow light" them. We also don't need to eat exclusively alkaline foods; we simply need to drastically reduce acid-forming foods and dramatically increase the alkaline-forming foods while we prevent food from sitting in the bowel. Then the problem will solve itself. I call this approach, "Starving the Yeast." It is a five-stage process that together starves off the yeast and bacteria that make our bodies problematic.

ALKALINE VS. ACID

My first memory of learning about alkaline vs. acid was in seventh grade science when we did experiments with litmus paper. A result of 7 was neutral; above 7 was alkaline; and below 7 was acidic. Well, our blood chemistry should be 7.4, which is slightly alkaline. There is no need to check it unless you're either very curious, or very sick. You will know if you are too acidic if you get sick often, get urinary tract infections, suffer from headaches, and have bad breath and body odor (when you do not use antiperspirant). Acidosis is the medical term for a blood alkalinity of less than 7.35. A normal reading is called homeostasis. It is not considered a disease; although in and of itself it is recognized as an indicator of disease. Your blood feeds your organs and tissues; so if your blood is acidic, your organs will suffer and your body will have to compensate for this imbalance somehow. We need to do all we can to keep our blood alkalinity high. The way to do this is to dramatically increase our intake of alkaline-rich elements like fresh, clean air; fresh, clean water; raw vegetables (particularly their juices); and sunlight, while drastically reducing our intake of and exposure to acid-forming substances: pollution, cigarettes, hard alcohol, white flour, white sugar, red meat, and coffee. By tipping the scales in the direction of alkalinity through alkaline diet and removal of acid waste through cleansing, an acidic body can become an alkaline one.

Bear in mind that some substances that are alkaline outside the body, like milk, are acidic to the body; meaning that they leave an acid residue in the tissues, just as many substances that are acidic outside the body, like lemons and ripe tomatoes, are alkaline and healing in the body and contribute to the body's critical alkaline reserve.

Starve the Yeast Stage # 1: Yellow-Light Starches and Sugars

Yes, starches and sugars feed yeast, but if you just drastically reduce the amount of starches and sugars in your diet and consume only the least offensive ones, you will immediately begin to starve the yeast that is throwing you out of whack. The goal is to starve the yeast by denying it the types and quantities of sugars and starches it was getting before, not by eliminating them entirely.

All grains other than millet are yeast feeders. Quinoa and buckwheat are next on the safe list of grains and may also be included in your diet. However, the best way to get your starch fix is through high-starch vegetables such as yams and winter squashes (pumpkin, butternut, acorn, etc.). These are really the only starches women should be consuming on a regular basis.

In terms of sweeteners, your choice should be stevia. It does not feed yeast. It is also natural. It comes from the stevia plant and has been around the health community for eons. It used to have an aftertaste that bothered some people, but in recent years, a company called NuNaturals has developed a formula that tastes great, so that's no longer a problem! If you haven't heard of stevia, it's probably because the sugar lobby would like to keep it a secret. (Not only is it all-natural; it has no calories.)

Unfortunately, all sugars (stevia is not a sugar) do feed yeast. Raw honey, agave, and pure maple syrup may otherwise be "healthy" sweeteners but they should be strictly limited on this program. Likewise, fruit, which is technically the healthiest food for the body in a cleansed state, will act as a yeast feeder before detox because of the high sugar content. Once the body is cleaner and back in a healthy balance, fruits and natural sweeteners can be enjoyed more liberally as long as the body responds well to them (meaning that yeast is not a problem).

The exception is low-sugar fruits, which can be included on the detox if desired. These include berries, Granny Smith apples, and grapefruits.

What Is Stevia and the Stevia Debate?

Native to subtropical and tropical South America and Central America, stevia is an herb extract from the plant *Stevia rebaundiana*. Estimated to be between two hundred and three hundred times sweeter than sugar, stevia has been widely used throughout Japan as a sweetener, and used as a dietary supplement for the treatment of blood glucose levels and alleviating high blood pressure. These beneficial medical factors, along with the fact that it is all natural, does not raise blood sugar, can be used by diabetics (and those on a carbohydrate-controlled diet), and contains zero calories, make it a very attractive alternative to sugar. It has enjoyed popularity in the health food community in the United States and Canada for many years.

Now that artificial sweeteners are no longer recognized as safe, stevia has entered the spotlight as a new alternative for no-calorie beverages and low calorie/low carbohydrate food products.

The World Health Organization recently approved the use of stevia as a safe food additive. This means that in the future all European countries will be allowed to use stevia extracts not only as a sweetener, but also as a flavor enhancer in many food applications. After reviewing many studies of reproductive and developmental toxicity with stevioside in rats, the committee of doctors and scientists reviewing the research found no evidence of steviocide being toxic or harmful to reproduction or development.

In October 2008 Australia and New Zealand's joint food authority (FSANZ) approved stevia for use as a food and beverage ingredient. In January 2009, Stevia was approved by the FDA with GRAS (generally recognized as safe) status.

I have enjoyed Stevia as my primary sweetener for at least ten years (through pregnancy and nursing two exceptionally healthy children). Coca-Cola and Pepsi are now hopping on the bandwagon with their own brands of stevia, called Truvia and Purevia, respectively.

Starve the Yeast Stage # 2:
Avoid Foods That Are Hard to Digest

Now that we have a better idea of what not to eat to starve the yeast, let's look at the next factor: avoiding foods that are hard to digest.

Nuts, grains, most dairy, red meat, and fruits all have a reactive, rather than calming, effect on the body. Nuts are extremely dense and difficult to digest, grains (with the above exceptions) are inflammatory, fruits feed yeast and cause a constipated woman to bloat, pasteurized cow's milk is highly acidic, mucus-forming and hard to digest, and meats are likewise highly acidic (as well as chock-full of hormones and antibiotics). It's the simple truth: **raw and cooked vegetables, avocados, raw goat cheese, organic eggs, and high-quality fish** are the main foods that support detox for today's woman.

Once a high degree of detoxification is achieved fruits, dried fruits, raw honey, agave, pure maple syrup, raw nuts, raw seeds, and high-quality grains can usually be integrated back into the diet with excellent results.

Dense fats are another barrier to cleansing. Women and fats don't get along well. Just when women were finally starting to get the message that oils and fats ought to be avoided, the raw food community comes out hailing the virtues of raw oils and coconut butter—some even promote the fiction that they can eat as much of it as they want and not gain weight! I quickly realized that by and large it was the men in the movement that were praising these fatty substances. Men metabolize fats much more easily; it's a more complex issue for women.

If you do still wish to use oils, be sure you are only using the cold-pressed, extra-virgin variety and only use them minimally. Do not cook with oils, as their molecular structure mutates causing cell damage and they become even more difficult to metabolize. When heated, even the highest-quality oils pour free radicals into the body. Real butter is a much better choice (women always look at me big-eyed with disbelief when I tell them this). Not only does butter retain its molecular structure at high heat, such as when sautéing or baking, but it is also less dense than oil. A pat of butter on a sweet potato or in a skillet for sautéing is absolutely fine. Use organic butter whenever possible as regular dairy is laden with hormones and antibiotics.

Starve the Yeast Stage # 3: Eat Quick-Exit Meals

The next part of starving bacteria requires creating what I call Quick-Exit meals. Remember, when food sits in the body it starts to fester. Even the best food will go bad sitting at 98.6° Fahrenheit for a couple of days. We need to prevent foods from remaining in the gut too long and the only way to do this is to create combinations that move as swiftly through the body as possible.

First you need to know which foods move very slowly through the system because they are so dense or gluey. We need to avoid Slow-Exit foods (these are also highly acid-forming), regardless of how they are combined:

Slow-Exit Foods

- Red meat

- Soy

- Processed foods

- White flour

- Cow dairy

- Nuts/seeds

- Beans

- Most grains (particularly refined grains)

Next, we need to avoid combinations of foods that create a slow transit. For example, fresh fish and sweet potatoes are both relatively quick exiters; however, when taken together in the same meal they create a very slow-exiting combo. Slow-Exit combinations are all meals or dishes that combine starches and fleshes in the same meal. Avoiding Slow-Exit foods and combinations makes all the difference in the world—especially for weight loss and increasing energy levels.

Quick-Exit foods are foods that move through the digestive tract quickly, giving the body what it needs and then moving out of the body. The longer a food or meal sits in the body, the greater the chance of it fermenting and/or putrefying. And when meals compile, this result naturally ensues. That's why we must make sure the foods we eat are "Quick-Exit-ors." It turns out that Quick-Exit foods are also calming, anti-inflammatory, and convenient. Here is a list of some common Quick-Exit foods that you'll be able to enjoy liberally. These are listed in a hierarchy from the quickest-exiting on down (least quick but still okay to consume):

Quick-Exit Foods (Note: with the exception of the animal products on this list, these are also the most alkaline-forming foods)

- Vegetable juices

- Raw vegetables

- Cooked vegetables

- Cooked starchy vegetables

- Millet, quinoa, and buckwheat (millet is a uniquely alkaline grain)

- Raw (unpasteurized) goat cheese

- Fresh eggs

- High-quality fish

Once you know what your Quick-Exit foods are you simply need to ensure that you combine these well so they become Quick-Exit combinations. On page 60 you'll find the Detox for Women Quick-Exit Combination Chart to guide you. But it comes down to a simple formula: flesh and vegetables *or* starch and vegetables.

Since the core foods on the program are the ones listed above, it will be very easy to create Quick-Exit combinations. The only starches included in the *Detox for Women* program are cooked, starchy vegetables (pumpkin, winter squash, sweet potatoes and yams), avocados, young coconuts, and a few grains (millet, quinoa, and buckwheat). These all combine with each other and with all vegetables (raw or cooked). In fact, that's exactly how you will combine these starches. They will not mix with anything else.

The fleshes that are included in the *Detox for Women* program include high-quality fish, raw goat and sheep products, and cage-free, organic eggs. (Some high-quality raw or pasteurized cow dairy is allowed now and then.) These fleshes also combine with raw vegetables of all sorts, as well as with low-starch cooked vegetables. (Not with cooked starches like the ones listed above or grain, avocado, or cooked peas, corn, or other cooked legumes.) Figuring out how to make Quick-Exit combinations is quite clear-cut. Flesh and vegetables, *or* starch and vegetables. Those are your choices at mealtime.

When you deviate from this approach, the slow-exiting nature of the food causes a domino effect that throws the body out of balance. We can deal with a few Slow-Exit meals now and then. But if too many start compiling, the symptoms and weight gain will start to snowball.

Starve the Yeast Stage # 4:
Create Space in Your GI (Gastrointestinal) Tract

Another element of Quick-Exit eating is creating space between meals so they do not compile. Limiting snacks to raw vegetables is a great way to do this. They are easy to digest and combine well with everything you'll be eating. The meals you do eat should be hearty and combined properly so you feel satiated and don't need to go around picking all day long.

To ensure that foods do not sit and that the body can make headway on the copious waste it needs to expel, two meals a day is all the food you want to take in.

One of the ill-advised habits we've culturally adopted is that of eating three meals a day (not to mention snacks). Not only is this too much matter for our intestine to break down, it overwhelms the bowel, which does not have the strength or the opportunity to work as it was designed to. When you eat the right amount of food—which is undereating in comparison with what the average person is used to consuming—you'll find your elimination is much more complete because your bowel can actually manage what you have put in it. It wants to do what it was designed for but it needs half a chance. Even women with a history of constipation are surprised by how quickly they start to have excellent eliminations once they are putting some space in their GI tract. And the key to accomplishing this goal is limiting solid food intake to two meals a day.

The best place to start is by cutting out breakfast. (Yes, you heard me right and I know this flies in the face of everything you've ever heard about right diet). Despite all the enthusiasm around breakfast, eating in the morning is not a health-generating practice. In the morning when the body's cycles are focused on eliminating what the rest from a night's sleep was able to process, breakfast is just too much food and too much density. When the body is asleep and resting from digestion it can do the work of processing new matter and awakening old matter for release, making some real headway on self-cleaning. That is why first thing in the morning people are at their stinkiest—their breath is bad, their tongues are coated, there's sleep in the eyes, and often odor on the body. This is the result of nature self-cleaning the moment there's a break from consuming food. This break from eating is essential. It allows the body to eliminate throughout the morning. The moment food enters the system, elimination grinds to a halt again because the stomach needs precious energy there to process the new matter.

The best scenario is to optimize the time between dinner and lunch the next day for maximum elimination effect. The way to do this is to avoid consuming anything requiring digestion in the morning. But there is something that you can take in that requires absolutely no digestive effort and will actually support your elimination as well as give you loads of energy: fresh, raw vegetable juice!

Your body may be used to the stimulation of cereal, eggs, raw granola, etc., but if you just give it a chance, you'll be amazed by how refreshingly delicious the juice is and how desirable juicing for breakfast can be—for your body and your palate!

Sunshine for Breakfast

Imagine eating sunshine. You do this when you consume raw, green leaves. Now, imagine drinking heaps of sunshine so that all that wattage of brilliant energy recharges your every cell. Imagine how you would glow with energy inside and out!

The diet and health community talks a lot about energy in foods; but the only real source of energy through comes from foods that carry the sun's energy—everything else is just false stimulation. All fruits and vegetables contain sun energy, but green leaves and grasses are actually synthesized sunlight. Chlorophyll is energy produced by photosynthesis (literally, "light change"). Sunlight changes into carbohydrates, which is energy that can be used by the body as fuel. Sunlight, water, and carbon dioxide all combine to perpetuate the life of the plant. When consumed, that energy enters into us to help perpetuate the life in our body.

Drinking the juice of green plants (romaine lettuce, spinach, collard greens, etc.) infuses the body with the sun's energy, renewing every cell it reaches. It cleans the blood through its rich alkalinity, near bio-identical makeup to hemoglobin, delivers the most absorbable form of minerals, floods the body with fresh Life Force Energy, and makes you feel absolutely fresh and energetic.

We have been led to believe that energy comes from calories or protein, bottled drinks, or packaged bars, but this is false. Energy comes from the pure animated electromagnetic current—the same source from which the sun gets the power and radiance that feeds us.

False stimulation, which can sometimes feel temporarily like energy (but leaves you crashing later), is what you get from non-sun food sources of carbohydrates, animal protein, and caffeine. The energy the body takes from chlorophyll is much more powerful.

The goal is simply to make the juices green but not super dark green—rather a blend of some light greens like romaine, celery, cucumber, and some dark leaves like kale, spinach, parsley, collards, etc. The more dark the greens, the more bitter and medicinal they are. We are not after a bitter, medicinal drink. Just because greens are good doesn't mean that the darker the green, the better. Very dark greens should always be balanced with light greens. Find a tasty balance of light and dark greens for optimum palatability and ease in the system. The Classic Green Lemonade recipe (page 103) is a good one to guide you.

A simple 50 percent carrot/50 percent romaine lettuce juice is another excellent choice and great for those on a tight budget or limited time. This is very inexpensive to make, requires minimal time and effort, and tastes delicious and refreshing. My clients and I agree that it's reminiscent of chocolate milk! My own juice of preference is a combination of some light and dark greens with lemon, stevia, and ginger. You'll find the recipes on pages 103–106.

While it's always ideal to drink juice immediately upon making it, you don't have to. If you seal it well and keep it cold, you can still have it a couple of hours later. For example, if you have to leave home very early, you can take it with you in a cooler and enjoy it throughout the morning. Another alternative is to make it and freeze it. Enzymes hold up pretty well when frozen, and if this makes it "doable" for you that's all that matters. So don't be swayed by those who insist the juice is useless unless you drink it immediately. There's much more to it than perfectly intact enzymes.

Make it tasty and convenient. Once you get into it you'll be hooked on the wonderful, clean feeling and energy it brings! Many of my coffee-drinking readers have reported losing any need for coffee when they have the Classic Green Lemonade. But if you still want your coffee, or are slowly transitioning away from coffee, you can have it thirty minutes on either side of the juice.

OVERCLEANSING

Overcleansing means more matter is awakened and loosened from the cells and tissues than the body's eliminative organs can manage to eliminate. When this happens symptoms like headaches, skin breakouts, excessive mucus, and even fever can result. The goal is to find a level of cleansing that is just right—where awakening is taking place but not so intensely that the awakened waste overwhelms the eliminative organs. This is why it is not wise to go headfirst into an all-raw diet or fasting program. If the waste is awakened but not released, it just makes you feel miserable, and then resettles in the tissue anyway rendering the whole attempt relatively futile.

This is also why so many people have emotional upheavals when they eat lots of raw food. All the old waste being awakened hits the nervous system, which runs through the middle of the colon. Then, it starts to go back into the body because the body wants to keep its center clear. This is not cleansing; this is self-poisoning. I'll say it again, "Detoxification only occurs when the waste *leaves*!!"

When waste is awakened and does not leave, it is a much worse scenario than if you had not roused the waste at all. In short, don't get caught up in the zeal of detox so much that you overcleanse. Pace yourself so that you consistently *awaken and release*.

Starve the Yeast Stage # 5:
The Grand Finale: the Food Waste Exits

Hurray! We won!

Once we are clear on how to stop feeding the problem we can move on to the actual detoxification part. Here is the key to understanding detoxification (it is missed by the majority of health and detox enthusiasts): **true detoxification only occurs when the waste residue sitting in the body (and the bacteria and yeast with it) leave the body**. Do you know how many people think taking a fiber supplement or a "detox" kit of herbs are cleansers? That's what these alternative health product manufacturers want you to think. But cleansing only occurs when a significant quantity of old waste leaves the body. Cleansing products and programs—like psyllium/bentonite products, raw food programs, and fasts are only *potential* cleansers. Unless the body passes the waste, it's not actually a cleanse.

Awaken and Release:
The Only Effective Detox Scenario

Effective detoxification is best accomplished by a method I like to call Awaken and Release.

When we eat alkaline foods we awaken the old waste matter. That's what putting real human food (alkaline, raw, water-containing plant food) on top of non-human food will do! But awakening the old matter is only part of the equation. The key to success is to *awaken and release*, loosen and remove! We don't want to awaken too much too quickly, so we must find the right balance between raw and cooked foods.

A good rule of thumb is to eat as raw and alkaline as possible during the daylight hours, which also ensures highest energy and productivity during the day, and then use the evening meal to slow down the cleanse to prevent overcleansing symptoms and offer pleasure, fullness, social ease, and emotional comfort. This is why cooked foods, fish, and so on, are recommended in the evening.

The reason women tend to get bloated when they start a detox is that they are successfully awakening the old matter but failing to release it. Men have less of a problem with this since they generally have more powerful bowels.

HERBAL CLEANSERS

Cleansing and regeneration come from the removal of accumulated waste matter from unfit foods and lifestyle. If you take one of the herbal cleanser "miracle" items and you wake up the next day with waste all over your body, pouring through your skin, or in the toilet, then by all means you've found yourself a cleanser. But I, for one, have not seen one of these. That's not to say that you cannot experience beginner's luck when you take an herbal laxative or psyllium the first time and have a great release. (Note: a great release is not liquid but actual matter.) That can happen, but it typically only works the first time because it is such a shock to the system. After that, these herbal laxatives only irritate the system and the psyllium fiber runs the risk of dangerously bloating and blocking the intestines. Psyllium absorbs ten times its weight in waste and if that waste doesn't leave the body—which it cannot do without a few good colonics—you will be *extremely* uncomfortable. I know it can be tempting to think you can just take a product that will pull all your past "sins" out of you in 48 hours, rather than undertaking the intelligent, longer-term cleansing process. These products seem cheaper than colon hydrotherapy and they promise to do the same thing. Herbal laxatives (cascara sagrada, senna, etc.) and chemical laxatives such as magnesium sulfate used to prep for colonoscopy can only clear a minute, narrow pathway in the intestine. They do not clean the colon. They just bring about a release of a significant amount of matter that makes people feel like they must be clean because they are not used to removing so much, and they are not aware of how much is actually accumulated in the layers of the intestinal walls.

Nothing can compare to the deep hydration and release that fully removes the matter from the layers of the intestinal walls, which can only be achieved with a series of well-administered gravity-method colon hydrotherapy sessions.

How Ladylike!

Now we have to bring up an "unladylike" subject. Alas, it must be done, ladies, or you will not smell, look, or feel very ladylike. This is the matter of bowel cleansing.

On this program, much more waste than ever before should naturally be leaving your system. The great thing about this approach to cleansing is that because of the absence of fruits and the inclusion of cooked food in the evening you are not likely to experience overcleansing, which means that too much matter gets awakened to easily pass through the eliminative organs, causing the awakened waste to recirculate and become reabsorbed by the tissues.

For many of you who come from a background of chronic constipation and IBS, just going once a day will be a great event. The high water content and increased bowel strength will definitely have you eliminating well at least once each day. However, you must give your body every opportunity for these eliminations to occur. First, you must make time for them—first thing in the morning a healthy body always has a substantial bowel movement. In a healthy bowel there is no need to sit and wait for an elimination—rather there is a clear sense that it is on the way. If you do not get this clear sense right away, then take the time to sit yourself down on the toilet and mentally send the message to your colon that it is time for the exodus. Nine times out of ten that's all it takes. The bowel has an intelligence. In fact, in a 2005 article in the *New York Times* it was noted that the colon housed our "second brain." Don't underestimate the power of a little colon telepathy.

In addition to making the time to eliminate, you must position yourself for the most efficient elimination. This means placing your feet about 12" to 18" off the ground to properly align your rectum. The modern toilet places the body in a *sitting* position, which is not ideal for elimination. The body eliminates best in a *squatting* position. (Observe your cat or dog squat when it takes its next movement.) By raising the feet you can correct the alignment and make it as though you were squatting (without having to put your feet on the commode and actually squat) over the toilet.

One should have a solid movement for every meal taken. So, if you are consuming two solid meals a day, you should find yourself eliminating twice a day (or having some serious "twofers").

If you are doing everything right and you are not having great eliminations, you might want to consider giving yourself an enema. Properly administered home enemas are completely safe and easy. I'm a fan of the Cara brand enema kit. This is a simple enema bag requiring nothing more than pure water and a bar to hang it from. Here's how it's done:

- Hang the full enema bag (filled with pure water) three to four feet above the ground. (The bath towel rack is usually at a perfect height for this!)

- Lie on your left side. Apply a bit of lubrication to the tip of the speculum (coconut butter works great), then slip the tip of the plastic speculum into your rectum. It only goes in about 1 to 2 centimeters deep.

- Release the flow valve so the water starts to flow from the bag, through the tube, and into your rectum. You will feel the water enter your body.

- Allow the water to continue to enter while you can comfortably take more. Once you feel you've taken enough water (the first "fill" or two may be short if matter is sitting down low, ready to release), clamp the valve shut. Sit on the toilet with feet raised as per a normal movement for optimal rectal alignment and allow the release. Ideally, matter should leave with the dirty water.

- Continue to fill and release as long as matter continues to leave the body.

- You should feel a charge of good vibes after a well-administered enema. The life force should feel like it is flowing in a strong current bringing a sense of undeniable well-being to the body and mind.

If you have access to gravity-method colon therapy and are open to the idea of having such a treatment, then you will be able to more rapidly achieve much greater levels of health, weight loss, and well-being than the diet alone can accomplish. If this diet-lifestyle is a quantum leap in the right direction, coupling it with regular gravity colonics is a quantum leap to the nth degree! Not everyone is geographically, mentally, or financially in a position to take advantage of this treatment, but if you are, or if you are creative enough to find a way to engage in it, I could not recommend doing so more emphatically. For a listing of colon therapists offering the gravity method, visit DetoxTheWorld.com.

Often women will say, "I'm afraid to cleanse my bowels or take on a cleansing diet because I go to the bathroom constantly." They feel they are not constipated, yet what they are experiencing *is*, in fact, constipation. Being constipated means that the heavy matter from the foods you eat is not leaving your system. When nothing comes out, or dark water comes out, or loose matter or a combination of ill-formed stools is all you are eliminating, those are all various forms of constipation. When you regularly see loose or ill-formed stools, you are constipated. This requires attention to bowel cleansing and cleansing diet as much as someone who is a "textbook constipation" case (who just goes very rarely or not at all). Soft, thick, heavy stools that make a hearty pile in the toilet are not to be confused with this—that's referred to as "cow plop," which is a good thing. There must be density to the movements to ensure that real matter from the food you are eating is leaving the body. Otherwise you are holding that matter in your system.

Additional Tools for Fighting Yeast and Building Up Armies of Good Bacteria

Probiotics are the good bacteria that help break down and eliminate the waste matter in the intestine. Since the modern woman's intestinal terrain is generally unfavorable to maintaining good bacteria, it is advisable to take these good bacteria in supplement form until the ideal good bacteria balance is reached. (A healthy intestine maintains a ratio of approximately 85 percent good bacteria to 15 percent bad bacteria. In modern adults it is usually the reverse ratio that causes myriad intestinal woes). Unfortunately, most probiotics in normal capsules are destroyed by the stomach acids long before they reach the large intestine where they are most needed. For these beneficial bacteria to remain alive they must be encapsulated in a more protective shell. There are several brands that now offer these well-protected probiotics that use a pearlized capsule. In my experience the best brand is Dr. Ohhira's Probiotics 12 Plus blend. It can be found at most health food stores as well as on my website, DetoxTheWorld.com. Probiotics should be taken on an empty stomach.

MODERN FOOD: NECESSITY OR SILENT ADDICTION?

Food is not usually perceived as an addiction, but I call it "the silent addiction," because the real reason people eat what they choose to eat is because they are addicted to food.

The problem with being addicted to food is that unlike other substance abuse, where you can distance yourself from drugs or alcohol forever, food is a part of every day. You cannot distance yourself from eating for very long. The kinds of food we eat today have become the great silent addiction. Like an addict, you think you will function better when you have your poison than when you abstain. Coffee addicts function best when they drink coffee, cocaine addicts function best when they snort, and Americans in general think they function best as long as they keep stuffing themselves with their poisonous food.

You may ask, "If 'normal' food is so bad, why is it that when people eat it they feel better?" Or, "Why do people who don't eat these foods usually seem fine?" Well, take away their coffee, alcohol, Prozac, cigarettes, painkillers, sugars, and starches and see how fine they are. They appear fine as long as they get their drugs. But like any drug addict, watch them try to function normally without it! It is not because the food they are eating is healthy; it's because the ingredients give them a fake energy.

Once people realize that their eating habits are also driven by a chemical addiction, it becomes much easier for them to master control and restraint.

Candex is a supplement that attacks the fiberous cell wall of yeast. The idea is that it incapacitates the yeast/fungus by destroying the outer cell wall where most of its weight is concentrated. Be sure to take this on an empty stomach. Candex is available at most health food stores.

Candi-gone is another highly effective yeast-fighting product. It is a two-part formula of yeast-fighting herbs. It includes many powerful yeast killers such as oil of oregano, olive leaf extract, uva ursi, pau d'arco root bark, clove, and more. It can be found at most health food stores.

I would suggest taking either the Candex or the Candi-gone first and then switching to the other product, rather than using them both at the same time. If you are taking a probiotic such as the one by Dr. Ohhira, be sure to take it at a different time than the yeast fighters, as they could kill off the good bacteria in the probiotics. (Example: Take the probiotic before juicing and the yeast fighter before lunch.)

Raw garlic is one of nature's classic antifungal soldiers. One clove a day of raw garlic sliced or diced into your raw salad is an easy and delicious way to help keep yeast and fungus at bay.

Step #2: Make a Plan

One of my favorite things about *Detox for Women* is that the program is convenient and easy. I should know—I live this way! But some of my clients are a little intimidated when they first hear about it. This is just a different way of eating, but different, in this case, doesn't mean difficult, even though at first it seems like a lot of new information. Don't write anything off as being too difficult until you've given it a chance (or you may miss out on the best part of your life).

Making things easy and convenient starts with having a plan. Since there are a few things you'll need, such as fresh juice and adequate produce for salads, you'll also need to have a clear plan to ensure you get these things. Your plan must factor in how you will get your food items and make your juice; how you will make sure you get the food you need at the office, when you travel, and so on; as well as how you will structure your days until you have this new way of living down pat.

Day 1 of the 30-day program is a perfect example of how an ideal day would be structured. Know your goal, see it in your mind's eye, and then plan ahead to make the vision a reality. This is the way all successful people get things done. You cannot achieve something if you do not plan it out.

Next you need to experience how delicious the food itself can be. That's when I know you'll be fully won over! So let's now take a look at what you'll actually be eating. It's much more satisfying and convenient than you might have presumed.

MORNING

The vegetable juice you'll be consuming in the morning is the only thing you'll have to go to a real effort to make or buy. The Breville juicer will be your only appliance expense if you choose to make it yourself (if you don't have an organic juice bar near you). The classic model Breville Fountain Juicer is priced around $150 (also available through DetoxTheWorld.com). The juice itself can be as simple or complex as you want to make it. There are many other juicers on the market but this one tops the list for ease of use, ease of cleaning, price, and facility of juicing greens.

Moving on to meal times: Since your daytime eating is going to be lighter than the evening meals, let's discuss your options to include the cleanest options first and then the options if you need or want to "bend" in the daytime.

NOON

The most detox-friendly lunch would be a large, raw vegetable salad with a green leafy base (mesclun, baby romaine, spinach, arugula, etc.). Add any raw vegetables you please (carrots, tomatoes, bell peppers, celery, cucumber, sprouts, etc.). You can even include raw olives and raw corn if desired. Then you want to add a whole, ripe avocado to make your salad more filling and richly textured. If you dislike avocados, you may use several ounces of raw goat cheese instead.

The way to add avocado for best taste and fullness is to chop the avocado up finely and then smooth it through the salad making the salad really creamy. It should become what I would call a guacamole salad. Then add some stevia (optional) and lemon juice. The combination of **lemon** (acid), **stevia** (sweet), and **avocado** (fat) provides a perfectly balanced salad dressing. If you need more than this you can either couple it with some steamed vegetables, a baked sweet potato or a cooked or raw vegetable soup. You should feel very satisfied by the size and taste of your lunch while keeping it raw-vegetable-based and light. You will get more used to it and become more satisfied by it with every day you do it. In fact, former lunch foods will start to seem too dense, complex, and heavy for you to imagine going back to.

If you need to "bend" the diet further to suit a bigger appetite or a business lunch you could select from one of the following choices as well:

• The raw salad as mentioned above with goat cheese (preferably raw, unpasteurized) in which case *omit* the avocado. Many restaurants offer a Greek salad with feta and olives, which would work fine too, even if it's not goat cheese (and even if it is not raw). Your body will still respond well to this combination.

- A raw/green salad with a piece of grilled or baked fish with cooked vegetables

- A raw/green salad with eggs—either as an omelet or a Niçoise salad with tuna, eggs, and greens. These are easy restaurant and diner options. You can always get a plate of greens and a three- to four-egg omelet (use the whole egg, not egg substitute!).

Ideally, you will not eat again until dinner but I realize that this may be unrealistic for some of you who are used to snacking. In that case here are your options:

Have more of what you had for lunch. Make more or leave some of your lunch for later.

Raw vegetables are always safe to snack on. Keep your favorites at the office, or wherever you will be when the urge typically strikes. You can dip in salsa if you like.

Having another vegetable juice in the afternoon or just before dinner is an excellent choice, as it will further alkalinize your blood and contribute to your overall alkaline "reserve." It's also revivifying after a long day.

If you know you're going to have a flesh-based/cheese-based dinner, you can have some of the Raw Goat Cheese Cabbage Sandwiches (recipe on page 126) later on in the afternoon. These are delicious and satisfying. You can eat several of these.

EVENING

Dinners should be very simple, easy, and satisfying.

Start with a green salad (adding any raw vegetables you like). Having a green salad before your meal helps to favor an alkaline balance in the meal, and the vegetable fibers and enzymes help shepherd the cooked food through for best digestion.

Here are your dinner options from "cleanest" to biggest "bend."

Your favorite steamed vegetables topped with grated raw goat cheese or organic butter and sea salt and/or a high-quality marinara sauce (such as those by Seeds of Change, Muir Glen, or my personal favorite, Paesana brand marinara).

Your favorite fresh fish (grilled, steamed, baked, poached, or sautéed with organic butter, garlic, lemon, sea salt, etc.) served with unlimited steamed or lightly sautéed vegetables. When you sauté vegetables or fish, you may use a little organic butter. Do not use oil as even the highest quality raw oils mutate at high heat and become difficult to digest.

Baked starchy vegetables like sweet potato, butternut or acorn squash, pumpkin, or even regular Idaho potatoes if needed. While squashes and yams (sweet potatoes) are biochemically superior to white potatoes, all vegetables, including white potatoes, are better than grains (except for millet and quinoa). Try to stick to the other roots but, in a pinch, a salad with a baked potato and vegetables will do. Feel free to use a bit of butter (ideally organic if you can get it) and sea salt or any spices you enjoy such as Spike or Herbamare, or pumpkin pie spice—which is great on yams and winter squash—to make it all as gourmet and tasty as possible.

Cooked millet, quinoa, or buckwheat (kasha or soba noodles) with steamed vegetables. Buckwheat noodles (a.k.a. soba noodles) are delicious as part of a vegetable broth–based soup with vegetables. They also work well with vegetables and marinara sauce. There are several brands of pasta that use only quinoa grain, which can be used for dinner as well with lots of veggies. Millet is the only alkaline grain and is delicious topped with a bit of organic butter and sea salt, and served with piping hot, steamed vegetables.

The highest-quality organic, free-range poultry (chicken, eggs, etc.) you can find, served with well-prepared vegetables.

Grass-fed, organic meats with lots of raw leaves and cooked greens (spinach, broccoli, chard, etc.). This is the kind of meal you only want to have on the odd occasion. Land animals are highly acidic and red meat is hard to digest. Left to sit and break down in the relatively long intestinal track of humans at

98.6° Fahrenheit it will become a breeding ground for bacteria. So you can eat it from time to time if you generally follow the rules of this book, but don't abuse this option.

Make sure your meals are hearty, filling, and tasty and you will not feel like you are missing out on anything.

It is okay to have a little dark chocolate (68 percent cocoa content and higher) for dessert. Occasionally, some ice cream, particularly the goat's milk ice cream by Laloo's brand, which doesn't taste at all "goat-y" by the way, would be fine. Their Vanilla Snowflake and Dark Chocolate flavors are wonderful!

I'll always take a bar of dark chocolate with me if I go out in the evening, as it gives me that little something after dinner that hits the sweet, rich spot without sabotaging my efforts to stay internally clean!

You don't need to be a gourmet chef to make simple foods supertasty. You just need to know a few things about food preparation. All good restaurants do to make entrees taste good is use garlic, oil, salt, and sugars. If you cook your fish or vegetables with a little organic butter, garlic, sea salt, and stevia if you need sweetness added, you will make something as delicious as the best restaurants. Vegetables and salads that have been properly flavored are not the least bit dull.

This lifestyle is meant to be simple and the food tasty. But planning is a way to make detox downright easy. Planning will keep you on the path and make sure you'll do it. Everything will flow smoothly. Who doesn't want a life that flows smoothly!

YOU CAN "WINE" A LITTLE IF YOU LIKE!

Wine does have some sugars and because it is fermented it does contribute to yeast. However, in my experience, if women stick to the program, omitting the greatest offenders that contribute to yeast in their food: sugar (from all sources), grain, antibiotic- and hormone-laden flesh, milk, etc., and they are releasing their waste well through the increased bowel activity, wine can be enjoyed. This seems to please my female clients immensely. They tend to be okay with giving up pasta, fruit, and bagels if it means they can have fish, goat cheese, vegetables, chocolate, and *wine*! Do everything else right and you can have your wine—that's the way to look at it.

STEP #3: Do It!

Women need to get out of the mind-set of being either on or off a diet. There is one truly sustaining way to eat. That should be the directive around food all the time.

Just as studying now and then doesn't make you educated, and cleaning your house now and then doesn't give you an environment of dependable serenity, eating right occasionally will never free you of systemic imbalances, make inroads against deterioration, or develop physical integrity.

We need to look at creating a daily routine that is not so hard that you cannot sustain it, but serves the purpose of keeping you from slipping back into imbalances and excess weight.

Take a good look at yourself, and figure out what you're willing to do. We need to make friends with our limitations. For example, if you travel a lot you're going to have to plan and prepare ahead. If you love sweets and starches you need to find ways of making cooked root vegetables and high-quality grains (millet, quinoa, buckwheat) work for you. To bridge the transition, come up with new recipes for the items you have a hard time giving up, like cookies—make them with quinoa or buckwheat flour instead of wheat. If you eat out of boredom at night, then you need to have lots of harmless foods like organic carrots, beets, grape tomatoes, goat cheese, ingredients for big salads, and cooked veggies. That way if you overeat you're not going to get yourself in trouble. The trick is to change the food and then the habits change themselves (instead of the other way around).

In my experience, women like meals to last. So make things that you can eat in large quantities like great big salads and large plates of vegetables. You need to provide the right elements so that you're psychologically satisfied or you will invite trouble (i.e., snacking on the wrong things, falling off the wagon out of a sense of deprivation or boredom, miscombining, etc.).

If you fall off the wagon, just get right back into the swing of things as soon as you can. Don't waste time berating yourself. That will hurt more than it will help.

TRANSITION TIPS: PIZZA, CHINESE TAKEOUT, PUMPKIN PIE

One great way to make the transition to detox fare is to think of things you love and try to mimick them. Vegetables are great with a little tomato sauce and oregano—and taste a lot like pizza! As for Chinese takeout, plenty of that flavor already comes with vegetables—try ordering steamed vegetables and a little grilled fish; add some soy sauce, throw in some garlic, and see if it doesn't spike them up. So much of what we love about food is really about what we put *on* it. Be creative with condiments. Don't assume that mustard can only go on hot dogs. You might be surprised. That's the kind of thinking behind my Pumpkin Pie in a Bowl Revisited soup on page 112. And it's no wonder that so many of my clients love it! And don't assume that what you love in a dish is something you can't eat. A friend of mine who loves the Greek specialty moussaka was surprised to find that what she was really crazy about was not the lamb—it was the eggplant! This is often true with pasta—women are surprised to find it's really the sauce they love, which they can pour over cooked vegetables and top with goat cheese for complete satisfaction!

It's also great to eat big portions and make a dish really inviting with color, warmth, pretty plates, and good utensils. Candles, anyone?

Include other things you enjoy that make you feel happy and spoiled around this time, like old movies or extra naps, sleeping late, calling best friends you haven't spoken with, candle-lit dinners, massages, or long baths, so you equate this program with pleasure and happy things.

Just a Few Hard and Fast Rules

One thing I tell my clients, which seems to really help, is that some things need to be kept sacred. Juicing, for example is one of those things. You make the juice happen even if it means planning ahead, buying a juicer, or even freezing juice when necessary. Juicing is king and if you want to alkalinize the body and avoid food in the morning, you make it happen come rain, sleet, or snow. Juicing is *sacred!*

One common trap women who are mothers of young kids fall into is eating their children's food. They'll make their children a meal and "pick at" or finish off what their child leaves behind. The trap is usually a combination of not having an organized diet for themselves and playing the tape in their head from childhood that programmed them to believe food should "not go to waste." (It's going to go to waste anyway, as you now know.) Ladies, this is one of those sacred things. You don't finish your kids' plates! Unless they are eating your food with you—forks and fingers off! Eating only that which is intended for you is *sacred!* No picking!

Figure out what you need to "keep sacred" to keep yourself out of trouble and make that the rule. For the few clients I work with who come from a fast-food diet background or eat common packaged foods, I recommend they pretend that the fast-food chain they go to has burned to the ground. It's not really there and going there is simply *not an option*. I have clients imagine that regular grocery store packaged foods are like children's toys and as such would be like eating plastic and paint. It is not food. "Strike that from your list of options," I tell them! If we perceive something as an option it will be. If we don't, it won't be. We do not eat certain things—that is *sacred!*

Making sure the plan is as realistic as possible is another major tool for long-term success. If you need to make juice for a week and freeze it to ensure you get it everyday, then do that. Remember to make friends with your limitations! If you can only shop for groceries once a week, get lots of sweet potatoes and broccoli for steaming, and other vegetables that hold up well over the course of a week.

Create a Big-Picture Goal

One key to success with any great project is to keep the highest goal foremost in mind with lesser goals beneath it. For example, someone who wants to be successful in business is more likely to succeed when she has a big-picture goal of high integrity. Someone who creates a product or business that others will need and benefit from will do better than someone who sells something cynically, just to make money. Look around; it is a pattern that plays out over and over again.

The same holds true for our physical transformation. If we choose a high-integrity, big-picture goal such as a lifestyle that makes a beneficial impact on the planet and our family, we are going to be more inclined to succeed than if we just set a common, self-serving goal, such as losing a few pounds or getting in shape for an event. I think it's because the larger goal gives us a greater sense of commitment. We know in our hearts how important it is.

Having a larger vision will ensure that you do all the little things every day that create a lifestyle to support real, long-term health, weight loss, and high living standards—while leaving a smaller ecological footprint and showing a good example to others along the way. This is not a sociopolitical point at all. In my experience this is the way long-term health strides are made, and why some succeed where others do not. Your rewards will be multifold, have far reaching effects, and impact the healing of your whole environment while you benefit in all the small ways you desire.

DISCIPLINE AND PRACTICE

One of my clients recently emailed me asking, "Is there anything in particular that worked for you or have you always just been able to 'restrain' yourself?"

I laughed when I read this email because I was never what you'd call a very restrained person. I realize, looking back, that I simply practiced being disciplined with small things and developed the "discipline muscle," which anyone can do if they only try (and set themselves up for success). I thought about the things that have kept me on track all these years and I came up with the following: I wrote back, "I just always make sure I have my favorites for meals: raw cheese, beautiful veggies, and all the things that make them tasty—stevia, garlic, lemon juice, sea salt, great marinara sauce, natural butter. Of course having the dark chocolate and occasional glass of wine have been very helpful as well! Otherwise, some things just became sacred to me like daily veggie juice and raw salads as the focal point of my meals (well-dressed with fresh lemon and stevia, of course)!"

I've grown to be disciplined. It's something that develops as you practice—like a muscle. The payoff has been well worth it and the food is so great. But I've also learned that life is for other things too—like experiencing pure energy, which you cannot do when your body is digesting heavy meals.

Calm Your Inner Life

Women were not meant to be plugged in to a high-voltage circuit day in and day out. It's no surprise that the body begins to short circuit. If you are at the mercy of the hectic, haphazard stresses at your work or in your family environment, then you are compromising your true self. Life is about being authentically yourself—not a conduit for the crazy energies outside yourself that you soak up unconsciously. This will destroy your sense of peace every time. Start paying attention to this and you'll quickly catch on to what is really your energy and what you're merely absorbing from what's going on around you.

You know that feeling after a long day when it seems like you've had yourself plugged into an electrical socket? You feel mentally frazzled and internally shaken up, but it seems normal because it's the way it always is for you after a long day. Finding a way to disengage from this energy is essential. Otherwise the old triggers that drove you to eat the wrong things, eat too much, drink too much, or smoke too much will still be there.

Simply taking a hot soak in a bathtub, lying down on the bed and breathing, or enjoying a guided meditation (see recommended CDs on my website, DetoxTheWorld. com) are easy and highly effective ways of accomplishing this. Just taking twenty very deep, slow breaths before you venture into the kitchen will help ensure that you calm all the frazzled energy that would otherwise have you eating in the same manner that you're "vibing"—mindlessly and quickly. Even if you walk home to a house full of children and demands, there are things you can do. (See the ten biggest excuses women make on page 155 for tips to manage this scenario.)

One common pitfall so many people trying to eat healthier fall into is thinking that if they slip up a little, they may as well throw in the towel and eat everything. There is nothing worse you could do! If you make a few errors or overeat a bit, don't make things worse. Your damage is only as bad as how much you give your body to deal with. If you take a meal with a few miscombining errors and then decide you've blown it, then chow down on all sorts of other unfit foods and combinations, thinking you can just start over the next day, your body will have to contend with those compiled errors and it will take longer for you to get back on track. This is not about calories; it's about not overwhelming the digestive system and preventing the feeding and breeding of bacteria and yeast. If you chow down on all the wrong things, then you are setting up something that is not as easy to fix as just starting again tomorrow. Stop when you see yourself going off the rails. Don't make things worse. Be pleased with yourself if you can keep a less than ideal meal or day contained.

Here's how to set up the best scenario all the time:

Decide what you want to happen: for example, you want to avoid poor eating habits at an event.

Project yourself into various stages of the future until you see the consummation of your desire. Using the event example, imagine yourself passing up the passed hors d'oeuvres as you cradle your wineglass, munch on the crudités platter, olives, and sheep cheese, and enjoy conversation.

Honestly examine every possible obstacle that could stand in your way. Imagine the bread being passed, the chocolate cake being served, the busy waiters that may intimidate you just as you decide to approach to ask them for a steamed veggie plate or grilled fish, instead of the meat and potatoes they have prepared en masse.

Contemplate solutions to these obstacles and how you are going to negate or overcome them. Imagine asking a friendly waiter for a salad and vegetables and passing up the bread. Imagine yourself being mindful of your feelings and the others at the table instead of chewing and drinking out of boredom or mindlessness. Imagine disregarding the chocolate cake (and maybe pulling out your dark chocolate bar, nursing your wine, or enjoying some herbal tea instead).

Keep doing this until your goal is reached or, in case of this example, until you are confident that you can enter into such a situation that might otherwise have tripped you up, and participate on your terms without compromising your wishes.

How to Proceed with Your Diet
After the 4-Week Program

In four weeks you are going to be convinced that core dietary guidance of the *Detox for Women* program is the way modern women should be eating regularly. In four weeks you will have come a long way—looking better (shedding most of your excess weight, depending on your size) and feeling significantly more energized and clearer mentally. However, your potential for well-being and beauty will only have been tapped. The longer you eat and live this way, the better the effects will be. You will get leaner, more toned, more radiant; imbalances of all types will diminish, and you will become more empowered. Therefore, I highly recommend making this program your "home base" diet. With that as your foundation, after the 4-week program you could begin to modify the diet to open up more options for yourself in the following ways:

At this point you could start to incorporate fruit into your diet. The best way to incorporate fruit is to have it before you take in heavier food (salads, cooked veggies, flesh, starch, etc.)—before lunch, for example. If you wish to have it following (or instead of) your vegetable juice, periodically, that would work. You could alternatively enjoy your vegetable juice in the morning and then have a fruit lunch, followed by a salad later in the afternoon if the fruit is not enough for you. It really is best to follow the "light-to-heavy" rule with fruit and eat fruit after juice. You could put an apple or two into your green juice instead of stevia, if you like. Fruit truly is the cleanest food for the human body; as your body gets cleaner you'll find fruit satisfies and energizes you completely. However, if you still get puffy and do not eliminate when you eat it, or if you still suffer from blood sugar imbalances it is best to wait until your body is a little cleaner to play around with it too much.

If you would like to integrate grains into the diet, keep in mind that grains are not ideal human food (millet is the one pure exception), so I don't recommend ever making grains a focal point of your diet. But if you would like to enjoy some pasta once a week, or bread, or even cookies now and then, this is what I suggest:

- Only use the highest-quality grain products such as buckwheat, kamut, or spelt pasta.

- Breads should be of the sprouted-grain variety. (Alverado St. Bakery and Ezekiel are excellent brands and have a tremendous range of sprouted-grain items, from bagels to tortillas and burger buns.) Spelt and kamut rice cakes by Suzie's are very good with salads for lunch, as are the whole grain crackers by Ak-Mak.

- The only cereals I would entertain would be whole grain kamut-, spelt-, or amaranth-based cereals (some by Kashi, Health Valley, or Barbara's for kids can be incorporated). Check the ingredients to be sure there are no refined starches such as white rice, white flour, or potato starch. Never use cow milk or soy milk.

- Milk alternatives: I recommend using nut milks with cereal. Pacific brand almond milk is great. You can sweeten with stevia or a touch of agave nectar. I would not encourage cereals for breakfast, but following a salad for lunch or dinner or as an occasional snack if desired would be okay.

- The best time to do grains would be your dinner meal, but if properly combined and of the best quality (per above criteria), they can be done at midday with a large raw salad, or in the case of a vegetable-avocado sandwich, on the sprouted grain bread. This is still much cleaner than the average sandwich and, as long as yeasts are kept in check, is a perfectly good choice on the maintenance program.

Nuts, unless you are cracking them open one by one like a squirrel, are just too dense to be considered as part of a daily diet. You could definitely enjoy them from time to time, though. Here's how:

- Nuts do not mix with grains, avocados, cooked starches like baked sweet potatoes, flesh like fish or chicken, cheese—even goat cheese, or fresh fruit.

- Nuts only mix with vegetables and dried fruits.

- One way to enjoy nuts would be to make a big raw salad dressed with a raw tahini dressing (lemon, raw tahini paste, stevia, Nama Shoyu, and garlic per the recipe in my book *The Raw Food Detox Diet*) and then top it off with 2 to 3 ounces of your favorite raw nuts.

- Only consume nuts in their raw state—never pasteurized or roasted. Sprouted nuts digest somewhat better but are still not light enough to be consumed with regularity.

- One might ask why they have been recommended in my past books. They are a very useful transition tool for many people to get them off of lower-quality foods and bad combinations. This does not mean they are a health food, or that they are good for women who are toxic (because they are so dense), or that they will support a light feeling in a cleansed system. They will not. But they can be incorporated when desired to no ill effect when abiding by these rules.

In short, we maintain and perfect the body by keeping to the tenets of the 4-week program while offering more choice to prevent against eating ruts, boredom, or creating too much restriction.

RAW CONFUSION

The original intention of the raw food movement was to bring high-water-content plant food back into the diet because it contained Life Force Energy and enzymes that the standard diet lacked. Raw food's origin was rooted in recognizing the value of simple food and its potential to clean cells. There was never a rule that one must eat "100 percent raw" to be accepted into the "raw club." Today, raw has taken a gross misstep away from those original, pure tenets by focusing on dense food that is difficult to digest like nuts, seeds, and raw grains in even harder to digest combinations, as well as way too much fat in the form of coconut butter, oils, and sugars. Unfortunately, this generation of raw has become another fad approach to eating that misses the mark. Raw juices, fresh fruits, and vegetables are the true healers, but there is still plenty of room for high-quality, well-combined cooked food in your detox diet!

INTELLIGENT CLEANSING

Cooked foods and non-vegan foods are not the enemy; just as all raw or vegan foods are not fit for cleansing. It's not as "black-and-white" as raw vs. cooked, or vegan vs. meat eater. Intelligent cleansing is much more of a tapestry of what is good for our physiology, while also balanced for our emotions and yet also convenient for our lifestyle. Yes, raw fruits and vegetables are the purest food for man, but knowing what we know about women today, we know that a woman fed exclusively on raw fruits and vegetables would bloat up and awaken waste that she could not pass fully on her own, and possibly arouse symptoms that would make her terribly uncomfortable. Our bodies are more compromised and we have more addictions and social pressures around food. All of this must be tempered with what we know about cleansing for it to be of real, lasting effect. Including fish and goat cheese may not be pure foods but that's okay. We need less-than-pure foods to intelligently cleanse in today's world and in today's body.

When it comes to detoxification, cooked vegetables, fish, and raw cheeses can be much more helpful than the common raw or vegan diet for several reasons. (1) By incorporating some cooked and non-vegan foods, the body is prevented from overcleansing. The raw fruits and vegetables magnetize the acid waste out of the cells with their rich alkalinity, high enzyme content, and hydration. If we were to eat raw, water-containing fruits and vegetables exclusively at every meal we would be "awakening" copious amounts of waste at every meal. This would overwhelm the bowel and make detox an untenable experience riddled with cleansing symptoms and much reabsorbed waste. (When waste is not eliminated after a few days of awakening, it recirculates in the body and becomes reabsorbed into the tissues.) (2) These high-quality, non-raw-vegan choices are easier to digest than many raw-vegan foods, and (3) These foods provide enjoyment and stimulation without feeding yeast.

Cooked foods, which are usually shunned in detox and raw-diet programs, are actually a help and not a hindrance when cleansing. The cooked food helps slow the cleanse to the perfect degree for maximum waste elimination without reabsorption. I cannot count the number of raw food women who have come to me for help after months of trying to be all raw. The raw food propaganda out there is very alluring. But without intelligent transition and bowel cleansing, it is a disaster for women.

Real Woman: Jennifer Gonzalez, 25, New York, NY

"No one has ever spoken to me so clearly and methodically on health and diet as Natalia Rose. Finally, a structured diet plan that made perfect sense! No gibberish about vitamins A to Z, folic acid, omega-3 fatty acids, etc., etc. It's impossible to believe that she's a day over 28 years old, or that her svelte figure popped out two kids. Witnessing this hard evidence firsthand only confirmed that I had discovered the fountain of youth. Needless to say, I was instantly sold and the rest is history!

"I literally used to work my ass off. I would never miss my five-mile run every morning before work, sometimes as early as 4:30 a.m. if I couldn't sleep. I was always sleep-deprived, dreading this morning workout because worse yet would be the regret of sleeping through it. My body was beat up, but I worked through the pain, telling myself that working out was essential for good health, despite my deteriorating bones. My hips and ankles were in terrible shape and after running my first and last 5K in September, I knew I had to give up running altogether because I could barely walk! I was totally confused. Were the endorphins and weight loss really worth this unbearable pain? And my diet was equally painful as I tried to follow the latest of doctors' orders. My bland food staples included dry chicken breast, steamed vegetables, and plain fish. The only food I truly enjoyed was baked butternut squash. I completely cut out salt, bread, anything fried, and my favorite, dessert (so sad). All of the running and minimal eating resulted in the end of my menstrual cycle and an exhausted look. I had to use a glycolic acid face and body lotion to get a synthetic glow. In fact, I would completely break out if I went a week without it. As debilitating as all of this now sounds, I was convinced that I was the perfect image of health because I was doing everything right according to any health expert, and running until the verge of passing out was, apparently, quite admirable.

"My priorities and my diet quickly took a 180 overnight after Natalia entered my life. However, my raw food diet was not without any transitioning of sorts. Before going raw, diet fad mayhem had me believing I needed to eat five small meals a day to keep my metabolism up. I don't do small meals very well. A tease to my appetite, these small meals would only turn into unnecessary mini-feasts, encouraging harder workouts, and ultimately triggering a vicious cycle. I didn't want to deprive myself when transitioning to a raw diet, so I ate as much as I wanted between meals to satisfy my physical and emotional hunger throughout the day. That, and being able to eat as many raw snacks as desired after dinner, helped make the transition easy. In fact, I was enjoying this way of eating much better than my previous habits. A nutritionist was giving me free rein to overindulge in dessert—who could argue with that? I was not gaining any weight even though I wasn't working out. Granted, I didn't feel very strong, but aesthetically, I looked the same, which was all that mattered at the time.

"Aesthetics was definitely the primary motivator, but eventually took a back seat to my concern for preventative health measures. My biggest health fear had always been developing osteoporosis and arthritis like my grandmother. It pains me to watch her accomplish the simplest of tasks like getting up from the dinner table. I thought that years of sports and exercise, coupled with not drinking enough milk, wasn't helping my cause. Ever since I was little, my grandmother would attempt to feed me milk so that I wouldn't end up like her. I've always hated milk, unless it was hot and chocolate. Hearing that milk actually leeches calcium from your bones was the best heath news I'd heard all my life!

"I eventually incorporated everything Natalia suggested, from dry-brushing, rebounding, sweating, and inversions to yes, even colonics. My day now begins with a full body brushing, followed by 15 minutes on the rebounder. After a year sans menstruation, I finally got my period back after rebounding less than a week! My periods are now regular, lighter, and pain-free. For that reason alone, I will be rebounding every morning for the rest of my life. Not to mention, the buoyancy of the rebounder is much more pleasant than pounding the pavement every morning for 45 minutes. I drink a liter of water throughout the morning and run to the juice bar at 2 p.m. to have my liter of celery/dandelion/kale concoction—an acquired taste seemingly for my taste buds only.

"Salad is my dinner staple and I make sure to eat a huge raw salad before having anything else. My favorite consists of an entire 11-ounce box of Earthbound Farm's Organic Baby Romaine lettuce or Spring Mix smothered with one whole avocado, and tossed with one whole package of dulse and a clove of garlic. I may throw some dulse flakes on top of it to add a "Bacon Bits" texture. Salad varieties are endless and surprisingly tireless and I never imagined myself looking forward to eating a salad at the end of the day. Along with my salad, I'll have 2 to 3 pints of sweet Jersey grape tomatoes or other bite-size vegetables (baby carrots, snow peas, sugar snap peas). I prefer them on the small side because they offer the same emotional comfort as grazing on a bag of chips. I then have an entire baked butternut squash for dessert (an old time favorite!). By the time I'm finished, I feel completely full, my love for a salty/sweet combination satisfied, and not missing the food coma or junk food craving. Not worrying about calorie counting, fat grams, saturated fat grams, good fat, bad fat, cholesterol, protein, sugars, or fiber, especially after a long day at work, is refreshingly liberating.

"I am secure in my body image and future health, a priceless feat. I can't remember the last time I got the tired, or light-headed feeling from standing up too quickly, both of which used to happen all the time. Most shocking of all, I've miraculously become a morning person! I attribute that to a rested body, the result of a clean diet. I am honored to share my story and hope that Natalia continues to inspire and educate both men and women globally now and forever."

part three

THE DETOX
FOR WOMEN
PROGRAM

The Programs

In addition to the core *Detox for Women* program, I have designed two adaptations on the classic program for you to follow if you think they are more appropriate for your needs. Most likely, you'll know which program is best for you right off the bat. Following the program descriptions are a few questions that will help you determine which one is truly designed for you.

The Classic Detox for Women: This is the core program. I use it with the majority of my female clients. It gets them into their best possible shape.

Adaptation #1: Baptism by Sunshine: This program was designed for those women who know that without a little bit of extra choice they will not be able to do this program. They are most welcome and should not be intimidated, but rather encouraged to do as much as they can with room to bend. The sunshine of well-being is let into their space so they can start to look and feel much better without feeling stressed beyond their perceived limitations around food.

Adaptation #2: The Systemic Cleanse: This program is for women who know they have a systemic candida infestation. Systemic simply means that the infestation is not contained in the gut but has permeated the tissues and it circulates throughout the tissues and blood stream. The Systemic Cleanse is a more intensive program that omits even the occasional low-sugar fruit, permitted grain, or treats like wine and chocolate. If you need the severity of this level and wish to follow it for 1 to 4 weeks, then candidasis should be fully eradicated. If your condition is severe, gravity-method colon hydrotherapy would ideally accompany this eating program.

The Detox for Women Test

Take the test and determine which program is best for you:

1. **Do you suffer from more than two of the following conditions?** Eczema, acne, hives, inability to concentrate, depression, lupus, vaginal yeast infections, IBS, rectal itching, chronic fatigue?

If you've answered "yes," then you might consider undertaking 1 to 4 weeks of the systemic yeast cleanse and see how your symptoms improve. Once they start to improve, you may switch to the Classic Detox for Women program.

2. **Are you feeling overwhelmed by the information in this book? Knowing yourself and your inclinations as you do, are you quite certain that it will be too restrictive for you to stick with?**

If you've answered "yes" to the above, then you would do best starting on the Baptism by Sunshine program as long as you need to. If you've answered "yes" to both questions, I would recommend starting with the Baptism by Sunshine program anyway to get the hang of eating this way and then move toward the Classic Detox for Women program. Chances are you will starve off so much yeast and bacteria just by shifting your diet to this degree that you will heal without the extreme of the Systemic Cleanse.

3. **Do you feel like your life has been an uphill battle with your weight and energy despite doing everything common dieting has advocated (low carb, fat-free, portion control, exercise, etc.)?**

4. **Do you finally want to know what it feels like to be perfectly balanced in your body (and see what that looks like too)?**

If you've answered "yes" to the above two questions, then jump right in and let's do the Classic Detox for Women program together! You will see results in the first few days, and in one month you will have scaled the heights of what the female body can become—and it only gets better the longer you do it!

A word to our men (yes, we love the brotherhood too!): All men can do the classic program. There is a certain male body type that is becoming much more common today and is characterized by a tendency toward yeast and bacteria overgrowth. Doing this program does not mean that you are in any way less masculine. It just means that you'll have a slam dunk way of getting into shape that is light years beyond the diets suggested in the men's magazines!

I have a lot of male clients whom I put on this type of program. If you are a man who tends toward bloating or "puffiness," if you are prone to gassiness and mood swings, and if you are a man who tends to crave sweets and starches, you will find this will work for you on many levels to correct your imbalances and give you a seriously enviable physique for all those clean-celled, gorgeous women that know a healthy, highly conscious man is the best catch!

The Detox for Women Toolbox

WHAT TO EAT . . . AND NOT

The following chart, which I refer to as the "toolbox," is something I developed in my practice and use with my private clients. The role of this chart is to clearly diagram which foods should be emphasized in *Detox for Women*, and which should be de-emphasized (or strictly avoided).

The first two columns are foods that you *will be emphasizing*. These are your "go" foods—they have a green light all the way as long as they are properly combined (as they are in the 30-day program starting on page 74). As the term suggests, the Hog Wild category lists foods that you can eat in unlimited quantities. I created the OK

Daily category for those foods that can be enjoyed heartily, but that I would not go so far as to say can be done in unlimited quantities. There should be some attention to portion in the OK Daily category without being too restrictive.

For example, since we're not mixing starches with flesh, one could certainly enjoy two yams or sweet potatoes with their raw veggie salad and steamed vegetables. Alternatively, one could enjoy a large piece of fish or several ounces of the raw goat cheese. (I'll usually eat the whole block of Alta Dena raw goat cheese, which is 6 ounces, with a raw salad for dinner.) This is not "portion control," per se, but these OK Daily foods do have a limit. For example, you would not want to eat two blocks of the cheese; or for that matter, a whole block of cheese and a big piece of fish, and a big salad, vegetables, a bar of dark chocolate, etc. That would obviously be *too* much food for your poor system.

The idea is that with the OK Daily foods, you enjoy them to satisfaction and exercise your good judgment without having to weigh, measure, or watch every bite you take. Don't forget to properly combine foods and start with a raw vegetable salad. Try your best not to compromise on food combining.

The Avoid column speaks for itself: These are the foods that for the reasons we have explained should be strictly avoided. However, there are exceptions within the groups of Avoid foods which are detailed in the Exceptions column. For example, while grain in general is not advisable, millet, which is biochemically less offensive and less inclined to feed yeast, would be fine when a grain dish is desired. Another example is in the case of fruit. While fruit should be avoided for the reasons we discussed, if the urge for fruit is strong, very low-sugar fruits, like the ones mentioned below, can be enjoyed from time to time during the program to no ill effect. I hope you find this toolbox as helpful and clear as others have. Take a moment to review it and notice how it incorporates all the knowledge we have covered so far and then hop down to the next section.

THE DETOX FOR WOMEN TOOLBOX			
EMPHASIZE		**DE-EMPAHSIZE**	
HOG WILD	**OK DAILY**	**AVOID**	**EXCEPTIONS**
All raw vegetables juices	Avocados	Grains	Grains (millet, quinoa, buckwheat)
All raw vegetables (including sea vegetables)	Raw goat cheese	Fruits	Low-sugar fruits (berries, Granny Smith apples, grapefruit)
Cooked non- and low-starch vegetables (spinach, carrots, beets, parsnips)	High starch veggies (sweet potatoes, acorn squash, butternut squash)	Nuts and seeds	
	Cage-free, organic eggs	Mainstream meats & poultry	
Lemon juice	Fresh fish (wild, organic)	Beans	
	Dark chocolate	White flour, processed and packaged foods.	
		Soy products	

As you can see, on the left are the two columns you'll focus on. Veggie juices, avocado salads, baked and steamed vegetables, and properly combined fish or starchy root vegetable meals will be spotlighted. The two columns on the right house the things you want to limit. This is the perfect portrait of how a modern woman should eat.

Now that you know what to eat, this table will tell you how to eat it.

THE DETOX FOR WOMEN QUICK-EXIT COMBINATION TABLE

This chart takes the foods that are permitted in this program and tells you which food category they belong to, so you can easily determine how to combine them to ensure they make a "Quick Exit" and do not stick in the body. Remember, both the starch foods and the flesh foods can be enjoyed with liberal amounts of vegetables, which are neutral.

Review this list until you are clear on what foods are considered a starch, a flesh, or a neutral item (notice how intuitively logical the classifications are). I recommend making several copies of this list to keep on hand (on your fridge, in your purse, at your office, etc.) to refer to until you have it down. Then, simply combine your meals such that the starches and fleshes never meet in the same meal or within three hours of each other.

STARCHES	FLESHES	NEUTRAL
Avocados*	Fish/seafood	All raw vegetables
Baked** starchy vegetables:	Raw goat and sheep cheeses (cow cheeses, preferably raw)	All low-starch cooked vegetables
Winter squash (acorn, butternut, etc.)	Organic, cage-free eggs (the whole egg, no egg substitutes)	Lemons
Yams		Stevia
Sweet potatoes	Organic, free-range chicken (if necessary)	Sea salt
Grains (millet, quinoa, buckwheat)	Grass-fed/hormone-free meats (if necessary)	Spices
*Technically, avocados are a fruit, but they combine as a starch for our purposes.		Wine
		Organic butter
		Dark chocolate
**In their raw, uncooked state they are neutral and may be treated as a low-starch vegetable.		Goat's milk ice cream***
		***However, it combines better with flesh, as sweet on starch can be gassy in some systems.

Note: All "starches" mix with other starches and all "fleshes" will mix with other fleshes. Netural items can be mixed with either starches or fleshes and may be enjoyed anytime with any foods.

Organics

Our farming and animal raising techniques are so compromised today that nothing is pure anymore. We "swim" in a sea of substances that attack our microbial health. Pesticides, radiation, and environmental estrogens (EEs) are just a few of the things that assault our cells and energy flow and imbalance our being every day. Nonetheless, we still have to make every effort to protect ourselves and this includes making every effort to use organic products and ingredients. True, it doesn't ensure purity but it certainly lessens harm.

The problem with the term *organic*, however, is that people have mistaken it as a catchall for "healthy." Organic only tells us how something is grown—it does not mean that something is healthy. For example, there's organic white flour, organic sugar, organic soy milk, organic coffee, organic macaroni and cheese made from organic white noodles, and organic powdered milk and sugar. So organic tells us something, but it's not enough to go on.

By the same token, you might be at a farmers market and find beautiful locally grown produce that is not organic, but you will enjoy it and you will create a cleansing meal around it. Don't avoid it just because it does not say "organic" on the label. Having produce from local soil is also helpful. But most of all, if you are just getting used to eating vegetable-based meals, having to concern yourself that every item of produce you buy is organic may be the straw that breaks the camel's back. Therefore eat organic intelligently—meaning, do the best you can but don't obsess. It is not the only factor. What typically happens as people get into this lifestyle is they upgrade their intake over time. Start with the right ingredients and the proper combinations and then step-by-step as you become cleaner and more sensitized to what you put into your body you will naturally gravitate to more wholesome, organically grown substances. Don't overwhelm yourself before you even get out of the gate!

Regarding Stimulants

ALCOHOL

All alcohol lowers the immunity of your body system. Beer is especially bad because it is made primarily with yeast and has sugar. Wine is also fermented using yeast, and it does contain some sugar, but this is the least offensive alcohol option, and may be included when everything else is attended to.

NICOTINE

Tobacco contains fungal residues, and it also robs the body of the oxygen which body cells require to fight the infection.

COFFEE AND TEA

Coffee and tea (even decaffeinated) have a negative effect on your adrenal glands. They put a strain on your immune system during a time when you want to give it all the support you can. If you must have some coffee, have it on an empty stomach (away from food), otherwise it will acidify everything it is taken with. The "civilized" after lunch or dinner coffee is one of the worst things you can do after eating. Herbal tea is fine anytime!

BEETS CAN TAKE THE HEAT!

Despite a reputation for being too sugary and starchy, carrots and beets are really very low in sugar and starch and rich in water and flavor! Baked beets are one of the best friends to a woman's bowel. I recommend baking the beets *in their skins*—don't even cut off the rough part on the bottom. Just rinse them and place them on a baking sheet at exactly 350° for 2 to 4 hours. Then either eat them hot or enjoy them after a night in the refrigerator—after which time they get sweeter and almost like they are caramelized. They are delicious, filling, and so good for the elimination! Don't be alarmed if you have a burgundy-colored movement (or a pinkish tinge to your urine) the next day—it's just the beets!

The Detox for Women Shopping List

REFRIGERATOR

Greens for salads: romaine lettuce, baby lettuces, spinach, etc.

Greens for juicing: kale, romaine, collard, spinach, dandelion, bok choy, watercress

Veggies for munching: carrots, tomatoes, cabbage, beets

Veggies for cooking: broccoli, zucchini, summer squash, spaghetti squash, asparagus, brussels sprouts, beets, etc. based on season

Raw goat cheese

Organic butter

Organic eggs from cage-free hens

Fresh wild fish (salmon, snapper, cod, trout, halibut)

FREEZER

Laloo's goat's milk ice cream

Frozen green juices for last-minute weekend or overnight trips (or when you're snowed in and can't get produce for juicing or make it to the juice bar for some reason). I keep a stash for all the above reasons.

COUNTER TOP

Starchy vegetables: sweet potatoes and yams, pumpkins, acorn squash

Avocado

Lemons

RAW GOAT CHEESE

As you know, pasteurized cow's milk products are not advisable, but goat's milk and sheep's milk products are fine—ideally raw but even the pasteurized goat products are pretty benign—like the soft goat cheese you'll get in a restaurant. Goat's milk and sheep's milk yogurts and kiefers are also great (ideally raw).

My favorite raw goat cheese brands are Alta Dena and Shiloh Farms. Alta Dena comes from the Alta Dena dairy in southern California. You can find out where it is carried near you at their website: altadenadairy.com. Shiloh Farms is based in New Holland, Pennsylvania; you can visit them online at shilohfarms.net. Note: Not all the items from these dairies are made from raw goat's milk. Always check the label and be sure that it says "raw" and "goat" or "sheep." Next best would be raw cow dairy and pasteurized goat or sheep dairy.

The best place to find these and other high-quality, organic, raw goat cheeses is at your local small health food store or farmers' market. Even if they don't have these brands, they probably have something like them. What makes this cheese special is that it's a hard cheese (jack/cheddar style) that you can use like any other cheese. Unlike the typical "smush" of goat cheese, you can slice it, grate it, or melt it over veggies. Kids, guys, and guests can't tell the difference (other than finding it delicious) because it doesn't even taste "goat-y." Even my lactose-intolerant clients generally have no reaction when they eat this cheese. It makes salads and veggies come alive; it makes a quick exit, and you can eat a fair amount of it! It's one of those things that I have to admit have helped me stay on the path for so long. If I know I can have cheese and still get to feel the way I get to feel and live life on such a high, what's there to complain about?!

CUPBOARD

Dark chocolate (brands: Rapunzel, Dagoba, Green & Black's, Endangered Species). Look for 68 percent or higher cocoa—some like it cold from the freezer, like me!

Stevia (brand: NuNaturals)

Herbal teas (brands: Yogi Tea, Traditional Medicinals, Tazo)

Marinara sauce (suggested brands: Seeds of Change, Muir Glen, and Paesana)

Nama Shoyu (raw soy sauce or tamari)

Sea vegetables (kelp, arame, kombu, hiziki)

Dijon mustard (suggested brands: Annie's and Westbrae)

Herbs and seasonings (basil, parsley, cilantro, garlic, onion, sea salt, pepper)

Millet

Soba (buckwheat) noodles

HANDBAGS

Stevia packets (or liquid vials)

Dark chocolate bars

Lemon and/or avocado and/or goat cheese (in case you're going somewhere questionable for a meal)

OFFICE

Lemons

Limes

Avocado

Packaged baby romaine lettuce or spinach

Dark chocolate

Stevia

Carrots or other vegetables for munching

Before we pull this information into a daily food plan, let's recap the goal that this diet seeks to achieve with the following effects:

1. Awaken the old waste matter

2. Starve yeast and bacteria

3. Rejuvenate the cells

4. Give the body a break from digestion so that it can put the energy into healing

5. Get enough food to satiate our hunger and desire for food without holding back the cleanse

6. Set aside time for relaxation and meditation to ensure your eating comes from a balanced, calm state

Now watch how it all comes together: Everything has been taken into careful consideration in creating the following program. As you know from the earlier chapters, there is a reason underpinning each moment in the day, so please try not to deviate too much from the basic program.

A Day in the Detox Life

"Okay, I'm out of bed—now what do I do?"

Nothing. First we give the body time to breathe. Then move. This is the best time to exercise. Rebounding first thing in the morning on a completely empty stomach is an ideal exercise for this lifestyle. Yoga, dance, or any other form of movement you prefer would certainly be fine as well. Try to take advantage of this moment of emptiness. What you used to perceive as a time of lack will start to be filled with the understanding that chi or Life Force Energy is another source of "food" for your body; as you stop needing caffeine or a heavy breakfast, you will start to feel really good, peaceful, energized, and clear at this time while your system is empty and quiet.

We have been conditioned to see emptiness as a bad thing—as something that needs to be filled with outside substances. Instead, as the body becomes balanced and the energy flows better, you will actually come to enjoy the emptiness and see it as a fine and pleasant thing to be used to your advantage as you make decisions about your day, and your life, as you stretch and move your body without liquids or foods moving around inside you.

Then, when the body has a call for something we start with:

Pure water: The first thing that goes into the body is always pure water. Despite the hydrating nature of the diet, we do need some pure water every day. Also, as a side note to the advanced students, we never put anything into the body until we need it. So we don't wake up and say, "It's 7 a.m., so I should have my breakfast—the rest of the world gets up and eats." That's social conditioning—not necessarily what the body wants. It's best to wait until the body sends out a call for nourishment. Even the most alkaline, enzyme-rich food can become acidifying if taken before the body wants it.

Vegetable juices: When the body calls for something more, we have vegetable juice. Don't worry, if you make it at home and then have it when you get to work, it lasts with strong enzymatic integrity even after it's made if it's kept well-sealed and cold. True, it will lose some vitality, but not enough to worry about. Also, keep in mind that the juice is important for more reasons than maximizing enzymes; it is there to provide a vitalizing substance to keep you feeling strong and satisfied as you abstain from digestion. It enables you to benefit from the power of a mini-juice fast each day. In terms of quantity, enjoy as much juice as you like! I recommend a minimum of 16 ounces, but you could have as much as 32 to 48 ounces to get you through the morning (and another glass or two again in the afternoon if you desire, but that's optional—like "extra credit"). Find the amount that works best for your body and your lifestyle.

If you require something more, aim for low-sugar fruits such as berries, grapefruit, or a green apple; but ideally stick with veggie juice or herbal tea sweetened with stevia. Your morning intake should be as light as possible. We're using the daylight hours to awaken waste through alkaline foods. The evening will offer more substantial food choices. So hang in there.

What about lunchtime? The morning was great but now I'm starting to get hungry.

Time to have your first meal of the day. Lunch will be a big, raw vegetable salad topped with a whole avocado. If this is not enough for you, or you're not quite ready for such a simple lunch, go ahead and add steamed vegetables and/or a baked sweet potato to this. (You can add organic butter and high-quality sea salt to your sweet potato or veggies if desired.) Lunch should be satisfying but not heavy.

Again, if you need more than this, or if you still feel the pressure of business lunches and the like, you could always have some fish or eggs—like an omelet with a salad. If you keep the combinations straight this won't get you into trouble. It's just nice to know it's an option since everyone is coming from a different physical, social, and emotional place—and we all find ourselves in situations that require a bit of flexibility sometimes. It's good to know how to bend without interrupting your progress.

It's 4 p.m. and I'm getting the munchies. What do I do?

You may still feel the habitual urge you to snack at this time for a while. Here are your best options:

> Some of you like to graze on small meals—for this, I recommend making a big portion and splitting it into two lunches—say one at 12 p.m. or 1 p.m. and then have the rest at 3 p.m. or 4 p.m.

Alternatively, you could enjoy something like the Pumpkin Pie in a Bowl Revisited soup (page 112), which is an all-time major hit! This makes a great cleansing afternoon snack.

You could have more veggie juice.

Raw veggies are always safe—you could dip them into a cleansing dipping sauce like a fresh guacamole or salsa.

Now I'm on my way home and definitely feeling stressed. How can I be sure I won't fall into my old patterns of eating tonight?

It's so true, a lot of women find it's easy to eat well during the day but when they come home it all falls apart. This happens for numerous reasons. The key reason is not hunger, but stress. You come home from your day—whether it's in an office, or with your kids, or in a classroom or hospital—and you've been absorbing other people's energy all day. We are like a sponge or a tuning fork—tuning into the vibration, absorbing the messages all around us. By the time we get home it's like we're carrying a caravan of other people's stuff in the door with us. This means we're not authentically ourselves at this point.

The only way to correct that is to break away from the inauthentic energy before we start taking it out on the kitchen. There are several things that work well:

Draw a warm bath and soak. You don't need any fancy stuff as water is good enough by itself. But you can certainly add beneficial herbs, or Epsom salts. What's important is that you self-soothe in the hot or warm water, breathe deeply, and let it all go. I manage to do this even with my kids in the house. When they were babies, I would just put them on the bath mat with a toy or a book. They loved the dim lighting and the sound of the water. They just want to be close to you. So many working mothers feel guilty after being away from their children all day; but they still haven't had a moment to themselves to collect their authentic rhythm. So taking a moment like this, even with them if you can, is a very important step to reclaiming yourself for the benefit of the whole. You could go for

---

THE WELL-DRESSED SALAD

A great salad dressing is simply the balanced combinations of flavors and textures of the following three elements: acid, fat, and sweet. All you have to do to create a wonderful balance of taste while adhering to these principles is combine the following in your salad: juice of a lemon or lime (that's the acid element); some stevia (I prefer the NuNaturals brand liquid stevia over the packets because I find the liquid blends better. That's your sweet element); and then for fat, you have your avocado. You'll see—it's so delicious! If you're a real foodie, you may wish to keep some sea salt and raw garlic on hand. This is really a fresh market feast and is so easy to make. You can use as few or as many ingredients as you like. It can be as simple as greens, tomatoes, avocado, and lemon—or complete with cilantro, garlic, and raw corn (which, by the way, is a vegetable until it's cooked, when it becomes a starch/legume). Enjoy fresh, raw corn on or off the cob—it can really make the meal!

---

a walk or a bike ride with older children. There's nothing more important than establishing peace within (which naturally becomes peace without) wherever and whenever possible. This will improve your family relationships, your mental clarity, your sleep, and have a hugely beneficial effect on your evening food and drink consumption.

Set your iPod to your favorite guided meditation: Doing a simple guided meditation before eating helps remove so much of the pressure that causes us to overconsume. One main reason people overeat is because they are eating while their brain is intensely spinning with all the thoughts from the day's experience and emotions. They are eating to the beat of their thinking rather than eating from a place of peace and clarity. A shift needs to occur to reground the body and become less polarized in the spinning head before eating. This will help prevent ill-consumption and overconsumption. Take the time to practice some form of meditation before the time of day when you typically binge or enjoy your big meal of the day, and you will find yourself eating much more slowly and registering when you have had enough. I have a list of my favorite guided meditations on my website: DetoxTheWorld.com. Note: I recommend lying down for maximum value. Lying down during meditation allows you to go into the deepest states, because no thought or effort is required to hold your body up or exert yourself in any way. Enjoy the experience of connecting with your pure essence. These meditations leave you feeling unburdened, refreshed, and enlightened, and improve sleep as they awaken your mind and heart for what is to come.

Thanks. I'm feeling more myself now. That really helped. I know I would have wound up bingeing or eating the wrong things with all that stale, crazy energy from my hectic day. It's good to be clear and feel whole. But I'm still hungry and cannot wait to eat! I have fresh veggies and other items from the shopping list in the kitchen. How should I proceed with dinner?

Dinner is the best part of the program. Let's get in the kitchen and start putting it all together!

You'll want to start your dinner with a raw salad. This is your "bulletproof vest," as my friend and colleague Gil Jacobs calls it. This salad will protect you from whatever cooked food comes after it. Your raw salad to start helps digest the cooked food, and fills you up on good stuff so you don't overeat on the less alkaline-forming, denser fare. Then you just need to decide if you're going to do a starch meal or a flesh-protein/raw cheese meal.

PROTEIN DINNERS

Even though dinnertime gives you a lot of leeway to enjoy cooked foods and animal products, it's important to start your dinner meal with a raw salad (even just a simple plate of green leaves). The alkalinity in the raw leaves and vegetables will help neutralize the acidity of those foods and escort them through the body more easily. You can choose from a wide variety of protein options, from eggs to fish to free-range chicken or even lamb, but just keep in mind that the lower-quality proteins are more likely to contains antibiotics and hormones.

I recommend anything from a raw veggie salad with raw goat cheese and fresh fish with steamed veggies to a raw salad with goat cheese and a pile of piping steamed veggies topped with marinara sauce and melted goat cheese. Again, it can be whatever you want in that category. There are recipes for this category on pages 136–142. There are loads of fish dishes, cooked vegetable dishes, salads, and cooked protein dishes that incorporate the goat cheese. There are also loads of root vegetable recipes.

STARCH DINNERS

These dinners will actually comfort your body and not just your taste buds!

If you want to do something in the starch category, keep in mind that the starchy root vegetables, like squashes and sweet potatoes, are the cleanest starches. Root vegetable starches are much easier on the body than grains—which is why they are emphasized, whereas grains are de-emphasized. Even regular white potatoes are "cleaner" biochemically than all grains (other than millet). They combine beautifully with avocados. So you could do a big, raw salad with avocado, like the Classic Daily Avocado Salad on page 123, with a couple of baked sweet potatoes, for example. More options are on pages 128–135.

You see, these dinners can be simple and clean while also being hearty and really delicious!

Be creative or be simple—suit yourself. There are enough recipes in the book and ideas you can come up with to create dishes you will love. For example, I always loved cheese sandwiches with tomatoes, mustard, and sprouts. Well, I don't eat grain, but I came up with the idea to take a cabbage leaf (green or purple) and layer it with thin slices of the cheddar-style raw goat cheese, tomato slices, Dijon mustard, and sprouts. I rolled it up and took a bite—bingo! It was exactly what I was craving. Now, I can have that taste whenever I want it and not compromise at all. Be creative with what you know!! While there's no need to alternate protein and starch dinners, I recommend limiting flesh intake to three times a week, as even the wild, organic fish is affected by the pollution of our waterways.

Excuse me, Natalia, I think you're forgetting one little thing . . .

I would never forget dessert! Are you kidding! I'll let you in on a little secret. I always have chocolate after dinner . . . my latest favorite (though they change all the time as I make new chocolate discoveries) is the Rapunzel brand with 70 percent cocoa.

For dessert, I recommend sticking with the dark chocolate. If you want to splurge a little, though, Laloo's is an excellent brand of goat's milk ice cream available at health food stores. While I don't recommend having it every day, it's great to have around (as long as you're the kind of person who can keep it in your freezer without eating the entire pint all at once). It's a wonderful treat to enjoy when the urge for a scoop of ice cream hits!

If you're at a restaurant and everyone is having dessert you could (1) bring your chocolate with you—bringing extra to share; (2) have a bite or two of a cream-based (not starchy) dessert like ice cream or crème brûlèe; (3) nurse your wine. Sometimes, I do all of the above. You could also have some herbal tea with stevia. Camomile or mint tea is nice after dinner, but you don't want too much liquid in the stomach after you eat, so sipping slowly is best.

30 Days of Detox for Women

DAY 1

> UPON RISING: Breathe deeply, body brush (see Body Brushing on page 78) and/or jump on your rebounder, stretch, do yoga—whatever movement makes you feel good. Wait until your body feels a need for something—never take food or drink into the body until there is a need. Then, drink one liter of pure water.

> LATER IN THE MORNING: When you feel the need for juice, prepare 16 to 30 ounces of Classic Green Lemonade (page 103). Enjoy as needed throughout the morning.

> OPTIONAL: herbal tea with stevia

> PRIOR TO LUNCH: any probiotic and anti-yeast supplements you plan on taking

> LUNCH: Fountain of Flavor Salad (page 118) with Raw Blended Carrot Revival (page 108), and baked beets

> AFTERNOON SNACK: Ideally, you will not eat again until dinner, but I realize that may be unrealistic for some of you who are programmed for snacking. In that case, here are your options:

> Have more of what you had for lunch. Make more or leave some of your lunch for later.

> Raw vegetables are always safe to snack on. Keep your favorites at the office or wherever you will be when the urge typically strikes. You can dip them in salsa if you like.

> Pumpkin Pie in a Bowl Revisited (page 112) or Raw Blended Carrot Revival (page 108) would be excellent choices for snacks. Just bear in mind that they contain avocado so be sure to keep this 3 hours away from cheese or flesh (as a 3:30 p.m. or 4:30 p.m. snack before a flesh dinner at 7:30 p.m. would be perfect).

Having another vegetable juice in the afternoon or just before dinner is an excellent choice, as it will further alkalinize your blood and contributes to your overall alkaline "reserve." It's also revivifying after a long day.

If you know you're going to have a flesh based/cheese based dinner, you could have some of the Raw Goat Cheese Cabbage Sandwiches (page 126) later on in the afternoon. These are delicious and satisfying. You could eat several of these.

Sometime before your dinner meal, either draw a bath or enjoy a guided meditation from the list on my website, DetoxTheWorld.com (or both if your lifestyle permits) to center yourself and release all inharmonious energies you may have taken on in the course of the day.

DINNER: Natalia's Favorite Salad (page 115) with Maple-Glazed Salmon (page 139), and steamed broccoli with organic butter and Celtic sea salt.

DESSERT: 2 to 4 ounces 68 percent cacao (or higher) dark chocolate is the best staple for everyday. Enjoy sipping herbal tea with stevia.

NOTE: 1 to 2 times a week include 3 to 4 ounces of Laloo's goat's milk ice cream

DAY 2

UPON RISING: Dry brush/rebound. Wait until your body feels a need for something. Then drink one liter of pure water.

LATER IN THE MORNING: When you feel the need for juice, prepare 16 to 30 ounces of Classic Green Lemonade (page 103). Enjoy as needed throughout the morning.

OPTIONAL: herbal tea with stevia

LUNCH: Life's a Rainbow Salad (page 119) with 1 avocado and 1 to 2 small baked sweet potatoes

AFTERNOON SNACK: Please refer to Day 1.

Sometime before dinner meal, take time to relax as described in Day 1.

DINNER: Classic Chopped Salad (page 116) and Raw Tomato Soup Topped with Shredded Raw Goat Cheese (page 114) with steamed greens.

DESSERT: Please refer to the directions given on Day 1.

DAY 3

UPON RISING: Wait until your body feels a need for something (never take food or drink into the body until there is a need). Then drink one liter of pure water.

LATER IN THE MORNING: When you feel the need for juice, prepare 16 to 30 ounces of Classic Green Lemonade (page 103). Enjoy as needed throughout the morning.

OPTIONAL: herbal tea with stevia

LUNCH: Guacamole Salad (page 124) and Pumpkin Pie in a Bowl Revisited (page 112)

AFTERNOON SNACK: Please refer to the instructions given on Day 1.

Sometime before your dinner meal, take time to relax as described on Day 1.

DINNER: Italian Salad (page 120) and Beet This Flounder! (page 136) with Cucumber Gazpacho (page 109)

DESSERT: Please refer to the directions given on Day 1.

DAY 4

UPON RISING: Wait until your body feels a need for something (never take food or drink into the body until there is a need). Then drink one liter of pure water.

LATER IN THE MORNING: When you feel the need for juice, prepare 16 to 30 ounces of Classic Green Lemonade (page 103). Enjoy as needed throughout the morning.

OPTIONAL: herbal tea with stevia

LUNCH: Classic Daily Avocado Salad (page 123) and Parsnip-Carrot-Beet Bake (page 133)

AFTERNOON SNACK: Please refer to the instructions given on Day 1.

Sometime before your dinner meal, take time to relax as described on Day 1.

DINNER: Green salad of choice and Raw Goat Cheese Cabbage Sandwich (page 126) with Detox Salsa (page 144)

DESSERT: Please refer to the directions given on Day 1.

DAY 5

UPON RISING: Wait until your body feels a need for something (never take food or drink into the body until there is a need). Then drink one liter of pure water.

LATER IN THE MORNING: When you feel the need for juice, prepare 16 to 30 ounces of Classic Green Lemonade (page 103). Enjoy as needed throughout the morning.

OPTIONAL: herbal tea with stevia

LUNCH: Quick Guacamole Salad (page 124), baby romaine lettuce, and 1 to 2 small baked sweet potatoes with organic butter

AFTERNOON SNACK: Please refer to the instructions given on Day 1.

Sometime before your dinner meal, take time to relax as described on Day 1.

DINNER: Life's a Rainbow Salad (page 119), Hungry-Girl Omelet (page 141), and steamed carrots with dill and organic butter.

DESSERT: Please refer to the directions given on Day 1.

BODY BRUSHING

Natural body brushing is a tool used for supporting the cleansing process by stimulating and releasing lymphatic waste. The proper method of body brushing is to brush the body starting from the tops of the feet in upward strokes toward the heart and lymphatic drainage centers in the body: the knees (backs and around the caps), the groin, and the armpits.

Using only a natural bristle body brush, which looks a bit like a horse brush (my favorite brand is Yerba Prima, available at most health food stores), stroke each area of the body two times toward the closest lymph center. For example, when you brush your legs, stroke each area as though you are shaving in upward strokes toward the knees, then on the thighs in upward strokes toward the groin. The backs of the legs and buttocks do not need to go toward the groin but they will receive a nice "lifting" of flow that will eventually improve the contour of that area. I recommend making circular strokes around on "saddlebags" or any areas plagued with cellulite. For the arms, start by stroking the palms of the hands to stimulate the reflexology points, then move to the tops of the hands and then, as you did with the legs, make long strokes up the arms (two strokes on each "strip") all toward the armpits.

The face, neck, and breasts do not need to be brushed—unless you choose to use a soft bristle brush just for those areas. Brushing the mid-section is good for digestive health. You can make clockwise circles with the brush to follow the natural movement of the colon: up the right side (ascending colon) across to the left (transverse colon) and then downward strokes along the left side (descending colon). A few circular sweeps will do. Then use your intuition to go back to any areas you feel may need a little extra attention, such as the sides of the thighs or buttocks. You may also brush your back if you like, but that is not essential. You should feel very energized and enjoy a clear sense of well-being after body brushing.

DAY 6

UPON RISING: Wait until your body feels a need for something (never take food or drink into the body until there is a need). Then drink one liter of pure water.

LATER IN THE MORNING: When you feel the need for juice, prepare 16 to 30 ounces of Classic Green Lemonade (page 103). Enjoy as needed throughout the morning.

OPTIONAL: herbal tea with stevia

LUNCH: Poolside and It's 80 Degrees Salad (page 122) Comforting Carrot– Sweet Potato Soup (page 108), and Avocado Wrap (page 146)

AFTERNOON SNACK: Please refer to the instructions given on Day 1.

Sometime before your dinner meal, take time to relax as described on Day 1.

DINNER: Green salad of choice, Maple-Glazed Salmon (page 139) and Simple Raw Sushi (page 131)

DESSERT: Please refer to the directions given on Day 1.

DAY 7

UPON RISING: Wait until your body feels a need for something (never take food or drink into the body until there is a need). Then drink one liter of pure water.

LATER IN THE MORNING: When you feel the need for juice, prepare 16 to 30 ounces of Classic Green Lemonade (page 103). Enjoy as needed throughout the morning.

OPTIONAL: herbal tea with stevia

LUNCH: Slim This Summer Salad (page 121) and Vegetable Soup Perfection (page 107)

AFTERNOON SNACK: Please refer to the instructions given on Day 1.

Sometime before your dinner meal, take time to relax as described on Day 1.

DINNER: Classic Chopped Salad (page 116), Herb-Encrusted Swordfish (page 138), Parsnip-Carrot-Beet Bake (page 133), and steamed greens.

DESSERT: Please refer to the directions given on Day 1.

DAY 8

UPON RISING: Wait until your body feels a need for something (never take food or drink into the body until there is a need). Then drink one liter of pure water.

LATER IN THE MORNING: When you feel the need for juice, prepare 16 to 30 ounces of Classic Green Lemonade (page 103). Enjoy as needed throughout the morning.

OPTIONAL: herbal tea with stevia

LUNCH: Fountain of Flavor Salad (page 118) and Pumpkin Pie in a Bowl Revisited (page 112)

AFTERNOON SNACK: Please refer to the instructions given on Day 1.

Sometime before your dinner meal, take time to relax as described on Day 1.

DINNER: Raw Caprese Salad (page 127), Simple Pasta Marinara (page 128), and steamed broccoli with organic butter and Celtic sea salt

DESSERT: Please refer to the directions given on Day 1.

DAY 9

UPON RISING: Wait until your body feels a need for something (never take food or drink into the body until there is a need). Then drink one liter of pure water.

LATER IN THE MORNING: When you feel the need for juice, prepare 16 to 30 ounces of Classic Green Lemonade (page 103). Enjoy as needed throughout the morning.

OPTIONAL: herbal tea with stevia

LUNCH: Classic Chopped Salad (page 116), Thai Delight (page 132), and Raw Blended Carrot Revival (page 108)

AFTERNOON SNACK: Please refer to the instructions given on Day 1.

Sometime before your dinner meal, take time to relax as described on Day 1.

DINNER: Quick Guacamole Salad (page 124), Sweet Butternut Heaven (page 133), and No-Fry Stir-Fry (page 135)

DESSERT: Please refer to the directions given on Day 1.

DAY 10

UPON RISING: Wait until your body feels a need for something (never take food or drink into the body until there is a need). Then drink one liter of pure water.

LATER IN THE MORNING: When you feel the need for juice, prepare 16 to 30 ounces of Classic Green Lemonade (page 103). Enjoy as needed throughout the morning.

OPTIONAL: herbal tea with stevia

LUNCH: Italian Salad (page 120), 1 to 2 small baked sweet potatoes and organic butter

or Thai-Flavored Carrot Soup (page 111)

AFTERNOON SNACK: Please refer to the instructions given on Day 1.

Sometime before your dinner meal, take time to relax as described on Day 1.

DINNER: Green salad of choice, Endive Bruschetta (page 125), and Kombu Melt (page 134)

DESSERT: Please refer to the directions given on Day 1.

DAY 11

UPON RISING: Wait until your body feels a need for something (never take food or drink into the body until there is a need). Then drink one liter of pure water.

LATER IN THE MORNING: When you feel the need for juice, prepare 16 to 30 ounces of Classic Green Lemonade (page 103). Enjoy as needed throughout the morning.

OPTIONAL: herbal tea with stevia

LUNCH: Life's a Rainbow Salad (page 119) topped with sliced avocado, and Gazpacho Means Summer Anytime! (page 110)

AFTERNOON SNACK: Please refer to the instructions given on Day 1.

Sometime before your dinner meal, take time to relax as described on Day 1.

DINNER: Natalia's Favorite Salad (page 115) and Simple Spiked Snapper (page 137)

DESSERT: Please refer to the directions given on Day 1.

DAY 12

UPON RISING: Wait until your body feels a need for something (never take food or drink into the body until there is a need). Then drink one liter of pure water.

LATER IN THE MORNING: When you feel the need for juice, prepare 16 to 30 ounces of Classic Green Lemonade (page 103). Enjoy as needed throughout the morning.

OPTIONAL: herbal tea with stevia

LUNCH: Green salad of choice, Raw Goat Cheese Cabbage Sandwich (page 126), and Detox Salsa (page 144)

AFTERNOON SNACK: Please refer to the instructions given on Day 1.

Sometime before your dinner meal, take time to relax as described on Day 1.

DINNER: Guacamole Salad (page 124), Parsnip-Carrot-Beet Bake (page 133), and sautéed baby spinach with crushed garlic

DESSERT: Please refer to the directions given on Day 1.

DAY 13

UPON RISING: Wait until your body feels a need for something (never take food or drink into the body until there is a need). Then drink one liter of pure water.

LATER IN THE MORNING: When you feel the need for juice, prepare 16 to 30 ounces of Classic Green Lemonade (page 103). Enjoy as needed throughout the morning.

OPTIONAL: herbal tea with stevia

LUNCH: Classic Chopped Salad (page 116), Avocado Wrap (page 146), baked beets and/or 1 medium baked sweet potato

AFTERNOON SNACK: Please refer to the instructions given on Day 1.

Sometime before your dinner meal, take time to relax as described on Day 1.

DINNER: Green salad and Maple-Glazed Salmon (page 139)

DESSERT: Please refer to the directions given on Day 1.

DAY 14

UPON RISING: Wait until your body feels a need for something (never take food or drink into the body until there is a need). Then drink one liter of pure water.

LATER IN THE MORNING: When you feel the need for juice, prepare 16 to 30 ounces of Classic Green Lemonade (page 103). Enjoy as needed throughout the morning.

OPTIONAL: herbal tea with stevia

LUNCH: Fountain of Flavor Salad (page 118) and Frittata al Fresco (page 142)

AFTERNOON SNACK: Please refer to the instructions given on Day 1.

Sometime before your dinner meal, take time to relax as described on Day 1.

DINNER: Fountain of Flavor Salad (page 118) and Grain-Free Asian Kombu Noodle Soup (page 113)

DESSERT: Please refer to the directions given on Day 1.

DAY 15

UPON RISING: Wait until your body feels a need for something (never take food or drink into the body until there is a need). Then drink one liter of pure water.

LATER IN THE MORNING: When you feel the need for juice, prepare 16 to 30 ounces of Classic Green Lemonade (page 103). Enjoy as needed throughout the morning.

OPTIONAL: herbal tea with stevia

LUNCH: Guacamole Salad (page 124), Sweet Butternut Heaven (page 133) and steamed greens

AFTERNOON SNACK: Please refer to the instructions given on Day 1.

Sometime before your dinner meal, take time to relax as described on Day 1.

DINNER: Italian Salad (page 120), Beet This Flounder! (page 136), and Cucumber Gazpacho (page 109)

DESSERT: Please refer to the directions given on Day 1.

DAY 16

UPON RISING: Wait until your body feels a need for something (never take food or drink into the body until there is a need). Then drink one liter of pure water.

LATER IN THE MORNING: When you feel the need for juice, prepare 16 to 30 ounces of Classic Green Lemonade (page 103). Enjoy as needed throughout the morning.

OPTIONAL: herbal tea with stevia

LUNCH: Slim This Summer Salad (page 121), baked sweet potatoes, and/or any other baked root vegetables

AFTERNOON SNACK: Please refer to the instructions given on Day 1.

Sometime before your dinner meal, take time to relax as described on Day 1.

DINNER: Life's a Rainbow Salad (page 119), Herb-Encrusted Swordfish (page 138), and sautéed zucchini and summer squash with fresh garlic and dill

DESSERT: Please refer to the directions given on Day 1.

DAY 17

UPON RISING: Wait until your body feels a need for something (never take food or drink into the body until there is a need). Then drink one liter of pure water.

LATER IN THE MORNING: When you feel the need for juice, prepare 16 to 30 ounces of Classic Green Lemonade (page 103). Enjoy as needed throughout the morning.

OPTIONAL: herbal tea with stevia

LUNCH: Guacamole (page 144) on baby romaine and Sweet Butternut Heaven (page 133)

AFTERNOON SNACK: Please refer to the instructions given on Day 1.

Sometime before your dinner meal, take time to relax as described on Day 1.

DINNER: Raw Caprese Salad (page 127), Simple Spiked Snapper (page 137), and steamed broccoli with organic butter and Celtic sea salt

DESSERT: Please refer to the directions given on Day 1.

DAY 18

UPON RISING: Wait until your body feels a need for something (never take food or drink into the body until there is a need). Then drink one liter of pure water.

LATER IN THE MORNING: When you feel the need for juice, prepare 16 to 30 ounces of Classic Green Lemonade (page 103). Enjoy as needed throughout the morning.

OPTIONAL: herbal tea with stevia

LUNCH: Italian Salad (page 120), Vegetable Soup Perfection (page 107), and steamed carrots with organic butter and dill

AFTERNOON SNACK: Please refer to the instructions given on Day 1.

Sometime before your dinner meal, take time to relax as described on Day 1.

DINNER: Green salad of choice, Has-to-Be Halibut (page 137), and baked spaghetti squash topped with Seeds of Change marinara sauce

DESSERT: Please refer to the directions given on Day 1.

DAY 19

UPON RISING: Wait until your body feels a need for something (never take food or drink into the body until there is a need). Then drink one liter of pure water.

LATER IN THE MORNING: When you feel the need for juice, prepare 16 to 30 ounces of Classic Green Lemonade (page 103). Enjoy as needed throughout the morning.

OPTIONAL: herbal tea with stevia

LUNCH: Classic Chopped Salad (page 116), Thai Delight (page 132), and baked root vegetables.

AFTERNOON SNACK: Please refer to the instructions given on Day 1.

Sometime before your dinner meal, take time to relax as described on Day 1.

DINNER: Green salad of choice, Endive Bruschetta (page 125), Kombu Melt (page 134)

DESSERT: Please refer to the directions given on Day 1.

DAY 20

UPON RISING: Wait until your body feels a need for something (never take food or drink into the body until there is a need). Then drink one liter of pure water.

LATER IN THE MORNING: When you feel the need for juice, prepare 16 to 30 ounces of Classic Green Lemonade (page 103). Enjoy as needed throughout the morning.

OPTIONAL: herbal tea with stevia

LUNCH: Classic Daily Avocado Salad (page 145) and roasted yams, beets, and parsnips cut into bite-size pieces and seasoned with fresh garlic and herbs as desired.

AFTERNOON SNACK: Please refer to the instructions given on Day 1.

Sometime before your dinner meal, take time to relax as described on Day 1.

DINNER: Hungry-Girl Omelet (page 141), Gazpacho Means Summer Anytime! (page 110) and fresh baby greens, and any cooked low-starch vegetables

DESSERT: Please refer to the directions given on Day 1.

DAY 21

UPON RISING: Wait until your body feels a need for something (never take food or drink into the body until there is a need). Then drink one liter of pure water.

LATER IN THE MORNING: When you feel the need for juice, prepare 16 to 30 ounces of Classic Green Lemonade (page 103). Enjoy as needed throughout the morning.

OPTIONAL: herbal tea with stevia

LUNCH: Quick Guacamole Salad (page 124) and 1 medium baked sweet potato with organic butter

AFTERNOON SNACK: Please refer to the instructions given on Day 1.

Sometime before your dinner meal, take time to relax as described on Day 1.

DINNER: Poolside and It's 80 Degrees Salad (page 122), Raw Tomato Soup Topped with Shredded Raw Goat Cheese (page 114), and your favorite low-starch steamed vegetables with organic butter and sea salt.

DESSERT: Please refer to the directions given on Day 1.

DAY 22

UPON RISING: Wait until your body feels a need for something (never take food or drink into the body until there is a need). Then drink one liter of pure water.

LATER IN THE MORNING: When you feel the need for juice, prepare 16 to 30 ounces of Classic Green Lemonade (page 103). Enjoy as needed throughout the morning.

OPTIONAL: herbal tea with stevia

LUNCH: Classic Chopped Salad (page 116), Thai Delight (page 132), or Raw Blended Carrot Revival (page 108)

AFTERNOON SNACK: Please refer to the instructions given on Day 1.

Sometime before your dinner meal, take time to relax as described on Day 1.

DINNER: Raw Caprese Salad (page 127), Simple Pasta Marinara (page 128), and sautéed green beans

DESSERT: Please refer to the directions given on Day 1.

DAY 23

UPON RISING: Wait until your body feels a need for something (never take food or drink into the body until there is a need). Then, drink one liter of pure water.

LATER IN THE MORNING: When you feel the need for juice, prepare 16 to 30 ounces of Classic Green Lemonade (page 103). Enjoy as needed throughout the morning.

OPTIONAL: herbal tea with stevia

LUNCH: Slim This Summer Salad (page 121) and Comforting Carrot–Sweet Potato Soup (page 108)

AFTERNOON SNACK: Please refer to the instructions given on Day 1.

Sometime before your dinner meal, take time to relax as described on Day 1.

DINNER: Quick Guacamole Salad (page 124), Sweet Butternut Heaven (page 133), and steamed broccoli with organic butter and Celtic sea salt

DESSERT: Please refer to the directions given on Day 1.

DAY 24

UPON RISING: Wait until your body feels a need for something (never take food or drink into the body until there is a need). Then drink one liter of pure water.

LATER IN THE MORNING: When you feel the need for juice, prepare 16 to 30 ounces of Classic Green Lemonade (page 103). Enjoy as needed throughout the morning.

OPTIONAL: herbal tea with stevia

LUNCH: Classic Chopped Salad (page 116), Avocado Wrap (page 146), and Parsnip-Carrot-Beet Bake (page 133)

AFTERNOON SNACK: Please refer to the instructions given on Day 1.

Sometime before your dinner meal, take time to relax as described on Day 1.

DINNER: Natalia's Favorite Salad (page 115) and No-Fry Stir-Fry (page 135)

DESSERT: Please refer to the directions given on Day 1.

DAY 25

UPON RISING: Wait until your body feels a need for something (never take food or drink into the body until there is a need). Then drink one liter of pure water.

LATER IN THE MORNING: When you feel the need for juice, prepare 16 to 30 ounces of Classic Green Lemonade (page 103). Enjoy as needed throughout the morning.

OPTIONAL: herbal tea with stevia

LUNCH: Fountain of Flavor Salad (page 118), Frittata al Fresco (page 142), and steamed carrots with organic butter and dill

AFTERNOON SNACK: Please refer to the instructions given on Day 1.

Sometime before your dinner meal, take time to relax as described on Day 1.

DINNER: Fountain of Flavor Salad (page 118), Sushi to Impress (page 130), and any cooked vegetables of choice.

DESSERT: Please refer to the directions given on Day 1.

DAY 26

UPON RISING: Wait until your body feels a need for something (never take food or drink into the body until there is a need). Then drink one liter of pure water.

LATER IN THE MORNING: When you feel the need for juice, prepare 16 to 30 ounces of Classic Green Lemonade (page 103). Enjoy as needed throughout the morning.

OPTIONAL: herbal tea with stevia

LUNCH: Natalia's Favorite Salad (page 115), Thai-Flavored Carrot Soup (page 111), and sautéed swiss chard with garlic and organic butter

AFTERNOON SNACK: Please refer to the instructions given on Day 1.

Sometime before your dinner meal, take time to relax as described on Day 1.

DINNER: Classic Daily Avocado Salad (page 145), Roasted yams, beets, and parsnips cut into bitesize pieces and seasoned with fresh garlic and herbs de provence

DESSERT: Please refer to the directions given on Day 1.

DAY 27

UPON RISING: Wait until your body feels a need for something (never take food or drink into the body until there is a need). Then drink one liter of pure water.

LATER IN THE MORNING: When you feel the need for juice, prepare 16 to 30 ounces of Classic Green Lemonade (page 103). Enjoy as needed throughout the morning.

OPTIONAL: herbal tea with stevia

LUNCH: Don't Lose Your Tacos (page 146) with a simple green salad

AFTERNOON SNACK: Please refer to the instructions given on Day 1.

Sometime before your dinner meal, take time to relax as described on Day 1.

DINNER: Baby romaine salad, Has-to-Be Halibut (page 137), and Grain-Free Asian Kombu Noodle Soup (page 113)

DESSERT: Please refer to the directions given on Day 1.

DAY 28

UPON RISING: Wait until your body feels a need for something (never take food or drink into the body until there is a need). Then drink one liter of pure water.

LATER IN THE MORNING: When you feel the need for juice, prepare 16 to 30 ounces of Classic Green Lemonade (page 103). Enjoy as needed throughout the morning.

OPTIONAL: herbal tea with stevia

LUNCH: Life's a Rainbow Salad (page 119) with Guacamole (page 144), Raw Blended Carrot Revival (page 108), and 1 medium baked sweet potato

AFTERNOON SNACK: Please refer to the instructions given on Day 1.

Sometime before your dinner meal, take time to relax as described on Day 1.

DINNER: Classic Chopped Salad (page 116), Raw Tomato Soup Topped with Shredded Raw Goat Cheese (page 114), and steamed greens

DESSERT: Please refer to the directions given on Day 1.

DAY 29

UPON RISING: Wait until your body feels a need for something (never take food or drink into the body until there is a need). Then drink one liter of pure water.

LATER IN THE MORNING: When you feel the need for juice, prepare 16 to 30 ounces of Classic Green Lemonade (page 103). Enjoy as needed throughout the morning.

OPTIONAL: herbal tea with stevia

LUNCH: Classic Daily Avocado Salad (page 145) and Parsnip-Carrot-Beet Bake (page 133)

AFTERNOON SNACK: Please refer to the instructions given on Day 1.

DINNER: Endive Bruschetta (page 125), Frittata al Fresco (page 142), and sautéed greens

DESSERT: Please refer to the directions given on Day 1.

DAY 30

UPON RISING: Wait until your body feels a need for something (never take food or drink into the body until there is a need). Then drink one liter of pure water.

LATER IN THE MORNING: When you feel the need for juice, prepare 16 to 30 ounces of Classic Green Lemonade (page 103). Enjoy as needed throughout the morning.

OPTIONAL: herbal tea with stevia

LUNCH: Fountain of Flavor Salad (page 118), Raw Blended Carrot Revival (page 108), and 1 medium baked sweet potato with organic butter

AFTERNOON SNACK: Please refer to the instructions given on Day 1.

Sometime before your dinner meal, take time to relax as described on Day 1.

DINNER: Green salad of choice and Maple-Glazed Salmon (page 139)

DESSERT: Please refer to the directions given on Day 1.

part four

THE RECIPES

Introduction to the Recipes

This recipe section was created with every woman in mind—from the woman who would rather not spend more than five minutes in the kitchen to the amateur and even professional chef. In fact, I've called upon one of my most cutting-edge chef friends, Matthew Boudreau of The Ram's Head Inn in Shelter Island, New York, to pepper this section with some of his interpretations on *Detox for Women* dishes.

You will see all the recipes you will need for the program here including vegetable juices, salads, soups, appetizers, and cooked dishes. All the recipes were designed to give you the most satisfying food experience, while allowing your body to release blockages. Detoxification through enjoyment of food is the way I like to look at it. I hope you enjoy these recipes as much as I do! Please note, some of the recipes in this section have been adapted from my previous books, per the considerations of the specifications of the *Detox for Women* program.

BETTER THAN A RESTAURANT—IN TASTE AND QUALITY!

When you consider the "raw materials" that go into the food a woman should eat—the ones that actually *belong in* and *serve* her body—you probably aren't thinking that you are supposed to like them. But well-executed salads and vegetables are fantastic! These recipes are not the typical garden salad in a mediocre restaurant. That, ladies, is not what I have in mind for you at all! I would not have been able to live this way with my penchant for delicious food if that were the case. I eat ambrosia when I make a salad. Even in restaurants, with a few squirts here and a few drops there, I can make the best tasting thing ever—the food of the gods!

To make salads and vegetables come alive we do not need thick dressings, oils, or heavy sauces—or need to thicken the dishes up with grains or tofu like you'll find in most vegetarian restaurants. Not by a long shot. Refreshing, comforting, soul-satisfying, well-balanced, fragrant—these are the terms I would use to describe the end result of a well-executed cleansing meal.

My Bag of Tricks

Although the following recipes will spell out exactly what you need for each preparation, I wanted to share my personal bag of tricks.

STEVIA

Clients often say that they don't use sweeteners. What they don't realize is that there is sugar in just about every product they consume—pasta sauce, dressing, soups, you name it. So while they may not *add* sweeteners, they enjoy these foods because they have balance of flavors that includes a sweet component. Since we've established that every sweetener other than stevia is unsuitable for today's overyeasted woman, stevia becomes a necessity for balancing dishes. Fortunately, it's easy to keep a small container in your purse, in your car, in your kitchen, even in your evening bag!

Stevia is completely natural and safe to use. It comes from the stevia plant and has been popular in the health market place for decades.

One of the most exciting discoveries I made with stevia is that when lemon juice and stevia are mixed there is absolutely no need at all for oil in a salad. This was an important discovery because on the one hand raw salads are the key to mealtime, and up until that point I thought I had to add some oil to make a salad tasty. Oils, as you know, are not an ideal ingredient for what we want to achieve. The oil is not needed to balance out the acid from the fresh lemon juice if there is a sweet. The sweet can do the same thing—particularly when there is already some avocado or raw goat cheese in the salad, which serves as a much lighter fat than oil. The flavor is worthy of full-out applause. I wish I could give you each a bowl of Natalia's Favorite Salad (a.k.a. "Lemon Cheesecake Salad") on page 115 (you can make it yourself and see) because you would know why this way of eating is so easy to maintain when this kind of big, refreshing, flavorful dish is center stage. The same is true for the Slim This Summer Salad and Guacamole Salad—and so many of the salads in the recipe section. You will find your own favorites and also find that you make them over and over again. That's fine! The idea is to find a few recipes that you *love* so you always have the ingredients on hand. That way you can keep your life simple and your taste buds satisfied.

COOKED VEGETABLES

Another craft I've taken for granted is that of cooking vegetables. I realized this recently when one of my clients asked me how I did it. I make vegetables the way a veteran knitter knits a sweater. It's so instinctual that I make the mistake of assuming everyone is going to know how to make cooked green leaves into the best side dish ever, or how to take all the vegetables that have accumulated in your kitchen that week and make them into a gourmet feast. It's not hard to do if you know how.

When cooking low-starch vegetables like summer squash, Brussels sprouts, okra, and greens (spinach, collards, chard, etc.) the trick is to heat a skillet on high with a pat of butter and a freshly chopped clove of garlic. Allow the garlic to absorb a bit of the butter and get brown (a minute or so). Next, toss the cleaned vegetables into the skillet (chopped in the case of non-green leaves) and let them mix with the garlic and butter (keep the mixture moving with a spatula to avoid sticking. Then gradually add a bit of water so the vegetables can stay in the skillet longer without adding more butter; and keep moving the veggies around for another 2 minutes, adding several dashes of high-quality sea salt.

Set the mixture to low heat, cover the skillet, and let that cook for about 3 more minutes; then shut off the heat completely, and either enjoy it right away, or let it sit a bit longer if you'd like it to stay warm until you're ready to eat it. The trick is the combination of butter, garlic, sea salt, and cooking.

Add herbs wherever possible. Some fresh rosemary, chives, sage, thyme, or cilantro all elevate the caliber of taste enormously!

Another other way to enjoy low-starch vegetables like the ones mentioned above is to steam them and then top them with a high-quality marinara sauce, like the ones by Seeds of Change, or my new personal favorite brand, Paesana. It's like having sumptuous, hot pasta. Top it with raw goat cheese for maximum flavor and you'll have the ultimate comfort food—something you and your body both crave.

The starchy vegetables like winter squashes and yams are best baked or roasted. These are so easy to prepare because you just throw them in the oven at 350°, leave them there for 45 minutes, and they are done. For roots with seeds, I recommend cutting them open, seeding them, and then placing them on a baking sheet with just a touch of butter and sea salt. Stevia can be used too and helps to bring the sweetness of the vegetable to the forefront of the palate. That's all there is to it!

The recipes are offered to inspire and guide you, but once you know how to mix foods and ingredients and the tricks, you can make any vegetable dishes and salads you dream up. As long as they adhere to the tenets of the program they will work. Delicious dreaming! Some of the recipes from my previous books have been revised to suit the principles of this program. So if you've enjoyed them you can keep on enjoying them!

THE SLOW FOOD MOVEMENT

I would like to draw your attention to a progressive movement afoot in the agricultural industry called Slow Food. Slow Food USA, founded in 1986 by Carlo Petrini, is a nonprofit organization that celebrates and rewards environmental sustainability, social justice, and the highest principles of taste and quality in produce, wines, cheeses, and livestock. It's "a food system that is good, clean, and fair." Slow Food is the opposite of the mainstream food industry. Its leaders realized how the industrialization of food was standardizing taste, and leading to the annihilation of thousands of food varieties and flavors. They wanted to remind consumers of their choices over fast-food and supermarket homogenization. The destructive effects of an industrial food system and a fast-lane lifestyle are clear, and we are invited by this inspiring movement to realize the benefits of a slower and more harmonious rhythm of life, starting with the cultivation of the fruits of our earth.

Herewith we have the preservation of taste, the support and protection of small growers, artisanal producers, and the physical environment. You can learn more about it at Slowfood.com.

Matthew Boudreau, executive chef and owner of Locavore, the highly regarded Ram's Head Inn restaurant, introduced me to the Slow Food movement. Here is a chef who grows many of his own ingredients and shops locally for the rich, local flavor. I love everything he puts in front of me, and begged him to share some of his recipes with you. You'll find them throughout the recipe section—and you'll find Matthew happily inventing and playing with local ingredients all summer long at his fantastic restaurant on Shelter Island, off the east end of Long Island, New York.

The Juices

All of the following juices are best taken on an empty stomach so they can bypass the digestive process and go right to the cellular level with all their life force and enzymatic superpowers!

natalia's classic "green lemonade" a la *detox for women*

makes 1 serving

> 1 head romaine lettuce or celery
>
> 5 to 6 stalks kale (any type)
>
> 1 to 2 packets of stevia or liquid Nu Naturals stevia drops (as needed for sweetness)
>
> 1 whole organic lemon (you don't have to peel it)
>
> 1 to 2 tablespoons fresh ginger (optional)

Process the vegetables through the juicer by admitting one vegetable at a time through the mouth of the juicer. The fiber will shoot out of the juicer into one container, while the spout will eject the fresh juice into another container. Pour into a large glass and drink! Notice how the lemon really cuts out the "green" taste that most people try to avoid.

life force energy power-ade

makes 3 to 4 cups

- 6 to 8 leaves fresh kale with stems
- 1 to 2 packets of stevia or liquid Nu Naturals stevia drops (as needed for sweetness)
- 1 whole lemon with peel
- 1 whole medium beet
- 1 head celery or 2 cucumbers
- 1 to 2 tablespoons fresh ginger (optional)

Put each ingredient one at a time through the mouth of a high-powered juicer. Pour the juice into a large glass and enjoy!

vegetable "chocolate milk"

makes 2 to 3 cups

- 1 head romaine lettuce
- 1 pound fresh carrots

Put each ingredient one at a time through the mouth of a high-powered juicer. Pour the juice into a large glass and enjoy!

Note: This juice is also great with a few drops of Nu Naturals chocolate-flavored stevia!

the great eliminator

makes 2 to 3 cups

1 medium or large beet
1 cucumber
½ to 1 head romaine lettuce
10 medium carrots
1 inch fresh ginger (optional)

Put each ingredient one at a time through the mouth of a high-powered juicer. Pour the juice into a large glass and enjoy!

the oxygenator

This elixir is great for increasing circulation. Enjoy the feeling of warmth as the ginger and chilies work to remove the blockages to your Life Force Energy. The beet will encourage bowel elimination and the sweetness of the carrots will soften the taste of the ginger and cayenne pepper, making for a smooth, pleasurable beverage.

makes about 2½ cups

1 pound carrots
1 medium beet
1 tablespoon fresh ginger
¼ teaspoon ground cayenne pepper or fresh serrano chili

Put each ingredient one at a time through the mouth of a high-powered juicer. Pour the juice into a large glass and enjoy!

green juice in a pinch

Enjoy only on an empty stomach.

I created this juice one day when I came home after a long day of work, feeling too exhausted even to wait for a delivery of fresh green vegetable juice from my local health food store. I remembered that I had some frozen wheatgrass cubes and whipped this number up. To my delight, it gave me the lift I needed and tasted great, too!

makes about 2 cups

4 cubes frozen organic wheatgrass (I use the Evergreen brand, which is available in the freezer at most health food stores)

1 to 2 bags of your favorite herbal tea (I recommend mint or orange)

3 packets stevia or Nu Naturals liquid stevia drops to taste

Juice of half a lemon

Place all of the ingredients in a large mug or glass. Pour 1½ cups of warm water (not hot) over the mixture. Let the frozen wheatgrass cubes melt, and then stir the mixture.

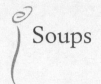 Soups

vegetable soup perfection

makes 4 servings

8 large carrots, chopped

5 stalks celery, chopped

1 leek, chopped

1 head broccoli, chopped

1 zucchini, chopped

1 cup mushrooms, chopped

1 cup okra, chopped

½ medium onion, chopped

Equal parts water and Pacific vegetable broth to cover vegetables (about 6 cups)

½ serrano chili (optional)

Spike to taste

Curry powder to taste

Celtic sea salt to taste

Place the carrots, celery, leek, broccoli, zucchini, mushrooms, okra, onion, (and any other vegetables you desire) into a large pot with the water, broth, chili, and spices. Bring the mixture to a boil and simmer until the carrots are semisoft. Best served with hot, sprouted grain toast with organic butter and/or raw honey. As with all homemade soups, the longer the vegetables soak in the water (even while in the refrigerator), the more flavorful the soup will become. For a thicker soup, you may blend half the mixture, then add it back to the batch.

comforting carrot–sweet potato soup

makes 4 servings

> 2 sweet potatoes
>
> 2 cups baby carrots
>
> 1 cup water
>
> 2 cups Pacific vegetable broth
>
> ½ teaspoon Celtic sea salt
>
> 1 packet stevia
>
> ¼ teaspoon cumin
>
> ½ teaspoon coriander powder
>
> ¼ teaspoon minced ginger
>
> ¼ teaspoon minced garlic

This soup is so easy (no chopping required). Bake the sweet potatoes and boil the carrots until soft. In a blender, mix all ingredients and process until uniform.

Pour mixture into large saucepan and heat to taste.

raw blended carrot revival

makes 4 servings

> 2 cups fresh carrot juice
>
> 1 ripe avocado
>
> 1 tablespoon curry powder
>
> 1 tablespoon fresh ginger
>
> 1 clove garlic

Blend all of the ingredients in a blender on high until smooth.

n pie in a bowl revisited

*is is among the recipes that I'm most excited to share with you. Why? Be-
ause this utterly delicious soup provides tons of live enzymes in an incredibly
digestible form. Neither my clients nor I can get enough of it. It's all raw, and
it supports weight loss and vitality, so enjoy as much of it as you like as part of
a meal or as a snack. I found that it's best to double the recipe when I plan on
having more than one or two guests. It may look like a lot, but this soup is so
good that you might eat most of it before your guests even arrive!*

makes 4 to 5 cups

32 ounces fresh carrot juice

1 cup raw sweet potato, peeled and cubed

1 to 2 packets stevia or drops of Nu Naturals liquid stevia to taste

½ avocado, pitted

½ teaspoon pumpkin pie spice

Place all of the ingredients in a high-speed blender and blend until smooth. Enjoy
right away or store in an airtight container and enjoy within 36 hours.

cucumber gazpacho

makes 4 servings

6 field-grown cucumbers, seeded and cut into rough slices

1 cup celery leaves and hearts, chopped finely

1 Vidalia onion, sliced thinly

1 jalapeño, seeded and chopped

2 cups picked basil leaves, ripped

1 cup flat parsley leaves, ripped

6 leaves of lemon verbena

4 ounces aged sherry vinegar

1 cup goat yogurt

Coarse sea salt to taste

Fresh black pepper to taste

Take all prepped ingredients and marinate together for 2 to 3 days in a plastic container. Place in blender and puree for 1 to 2 minutes—not too long as you don't
want the veggies to break down to a point of a watery base. Once you have a basic
puree of veggies, with no large chunks, mix in the yogurt by hand to get a creamy
consistency. If you like, add a little diced cucumber and grapeseed oil to the top of
the soup for garnish and texture.

gazpacho means summer anytime!

makes 4 servings

For the Soup Base

6 medium vine-ripe tomatoes, halved

½ to 1 cup packed fresh basil

⅓ cup fresh lemon juice

1 teaspoon Nama Shoyu soy sauce

1 clove garlic

1 to 2 teaspoons Spike

Celtic sea salt and freshly ground black pepper to taste

For the "Meat"

1 yellow bell pepper, finely chopped

1 to 2 ears fresh corn, kernels cut off the cob

¼ jicama, chopped

To make the base: In a blender, combine all of the ingredients and blend until desired consistency is reached. You may use the whole tomatoes, including skin and seeds.

For the "chunky" part: Combine the chopped vegetables in a large bowl. Pour the base mixture into the bowl and mix well. Serve well-chilled. It tastes even better the next day!

thai-flavored carrot soup

makes 4 servings

15 carrots, cut into 1- to 2-inch slices

32 ounces Pacific vegetable broth

2 tablespoons lemongrass

1 small Spanish onion, chopped

3 tablespoons curry (or to taste)

3 tablespoons Spike seasoning

1 tablespoon minced ginger

2 to 3 cloves garlic

Fresh cilantro

Place the carrots, broth, lemongrass, and onion into a soup pot. Bring to a boil simmer until the carrots are medium-soft (you should be able to pierce them with a fork). Let it cool. Put small batches (about 2 cups at a time) of the mixture into your blender and purée. Once it's all puréed, add the curry, Spike, ginger, and garlic until it suits your taste. Serve with fresh cilantro.

pumpk

grain-free asian kombu noodle soup

This is a great cold weather soup. It really heats you up inside.

makes about 5 cups or 4 servings

3 cups organic vegetable broth

1 cup carrots, julienned

1 cup lotus root, thinly sliced (optional)

1 cup shiitake mushrooms, sliced

1 tablespoon fresh ginger, minced

1 tablespoon fresh garlic, minced

1 tablespoon soy sauce (the Nama Shoyu brand, if possible)

2 packets soft Kombu seaweed noodles, rinsed (see note below)

½ cup snow pea shoots (available in most gourmet stores and farmers' markets, but if you cannot find them, they may be omitted)

In a large soup pot, combine all of the ingredients except the Kombu noodles and the snow pea shoots. Bring ingredients to a boil and let simmer for about 10 minutes. Ladle the soup mixture evenly on top of the Kombu noodles in a large serving bowl. Dress with the snow pea shoots.

Note: If you cannot find Kombu seaweed noodles easily at your health food or gourmet grocery, you may order them online at www.kombu-noodle.com. This particular brand is soft and pastalike, packed in water and ready to use.

raw tomato soup topped with shredded raw goat cheese

Bliss!

makes 2 servings

5 Roma or Holland tomatoes, diced

4 sun-dried tomatoes, soaked in warm water until soft and diced

¼ cup fresh basil leaves, chopped

1 clove garlic, diced

2 tablespoons fresh oregano, finely chopped

½ cup raw cheddar-style goat cheese, shredded (I recommend Alta Dena, but
   Shiloh Farms or any other brand will do)

Sea salt and fresh pepper to taste

In a large bowl, mix together all of the ingredients except the shredded cheese.
Distribute evenly into two soup bowls and top with the shredded cheese. Serve at
room temperature or slightly warmed.

Salads

natalia's favorite salad (a.k.a. lemon cheesecake salad)

This is the salad I eat more often than any other. I love the way the fresh lemon juice, stevia, and grated goat cheese come together so decadently, while the greens and tomatoes keep the whole dish tasting fresh from the garden. The beets offer a colorful twist, reminiscent of the great beet and goat cheese salads at the best French bistros. For a simpler dish, try this recipe without the optional herbs and onion. For a showpiece, add everything!

makes 2 to 4 servings

¼ to ½ pounds baby romaine lettuce or baby spinach (try mixing both together!)

½ cup of the best local tomatoes you can find, chopped

3 ounces Alta Dena raw cheddar-style goat cheese, grated

¼ cup fresh lemon juice

3 to 4 packets stevia or 1 teaspoon of the Nu Naturals liquid stevia drops 1 tablespoon fresh garlic, diced

Keep it as simple as the above list of ingredients if time and ingredients are constrained or make it really gourmet for a dinner party by adding the following:

2 tablespoons sweet onion, diced (optional)

¼ cup fresh basil, chopped (optional)

2 tablespoons fresh oregano, rosemary, or chives (or all three), chopped

Toss all of the ingredients together in a large salad bowl and serve (and serve and serve . . .)

classic chopped salad

makes 4 servings

1 cup fresh haricots verts (green beans)

3 ears fresh corn, kernels cut from cob

1 yellow bell pepper, chopped

2 large carrots, chopped

2 cups grape tomatoes, sliced in half

1 zucchini, chopped

3 tablespoons fresh chives, minced

¼ cup fresh lemon juice

Stevia to taste

1 teaspoon fresh garlic, diced

Mix all ingredients in a large bowl.

CLEANSING HAUTE CUISINE COURTESY OF
CHEF MATTHEW BOUDREAU

simple farmer's greens salad

makes 4 servings

6 cups farmers' market greens

1 cucumber, seeded and sliced paper thin

12 grape tomatoes, halved

6 radishes, quartered

1 cup flat parsley leaves, ripped

2 shallots, sliced paper-thin

8 ounces Catapano farm goat cheese

Lemon Truffle Vinaigrette

1 whole avocado, ripened

4 ounces fresh lemon juice

¼ teaspoon of cayenne pepper (optional)

Fine sea salt to taste

Fresh black pepper to taste

Prep all veggies and keep separate until ready to assemble.

Pit avocado and remove skin. In a bowl, mash the avocado, add lemon juice, mash with half the goat cheese, then season to taste. Take remainder of cheese and crumble on top. Enjoy.

fountain of flavor salad

Clove and cinnamon add wonderful elements of surprise to a dish. This salad warms your senses and triggers further creativity in the kitchen by mixing warm and tangy with a touch of Indian spice.

makes 4 servings

½ pound romaine lettuce, chopped (or ½ pound baby lettuces)

1 cup cherry tomatoes, sliced in half

1 teaspoon cinnamon

1 teaspoon ground cloves

1 clove garlic, chopped

1 ½ teaspoons fresh oregano, chopped

1 ½ teaspoons fresh thyme, chopped

2 tablespoons fresh lemon juice

Stevia powder or liquid drops to taste

4 raw olives, chopped

Celtic sea salt and freshly ground pepper to taste

Add all of the ingredients into a mixing bowl. Toss well and enjoy!

life's a rainbow salad

This is a simply beautiful creation that will appeal to everyone.

makes 2 to 4 servings

½ cup red cabbage, shredded or finely chopped

½ cup yellow bell pepper, julienned or chopped

½ cup carrots, shredded

½ cup alfalfa sprouts

1 cup mesclun greens or baby lettuces

¼ cup fresh lemon juice

Stevia to taste

1 teaspoon diced fresh garlic

Place the red cabbage, yellow peppers, carrots, and sprouts in little piles forming a circle around the greens like a rainbow. Mix the lemon juice, Stevia, and garlic and dress the vegetables.

italian salad

makes 2 to 4 servings

1 head romaine, chopped

2 cups arugula, chopped

2 yellow bell peppers, finely chopped

4 Roma tomatoes, chopped

4 sun-dried tomatoes, soaked and chopped

1 zucchini, julienned

¼ cup chopped fresh basil

1 tablespoon minced garlic

½ cup fresh lemon juice

Celtic sea salt and freshly ground black pepper to taste

Mix all the vegetables in a large bowl. Dress with the basil, garlic, lemon juice, sea salt, and pepper.

slim this summer salad

This recipe is the closest I have come to mimicking the flavor of pizza in a salad.

makes 2 servings

6 to 8 unsulfured sun-dried tomatoes, soaked in lukewarm water until soft,
   chopped

¼ to ½ pound fresh baby greens

3 ounces Alta Dena or Shiloh Farms raw cheddar-style goat cheese, shredded

¼ cup fresh chopped basil

1 tablespoon chopped oregano

1 tablespoon fresh lemon juice

2 packets stevia

1 clove garlic, chopped (optional)

Sea salt and pepper to taste

Mix all of the ingredients together and devour!

poolside and it's 80 degrees salad

makes 1 to 2 servings

    2 ounces fresh arugula or spinach

    1 avocado, sliced

    1 bulb fennel, julienned

    ½ cup sweet cherry tomatoes, halved

    1 orange bell pepper, julienned

    ¼ cup sliced scallions

    1 tablespoon fresh dill (optional)

    1 tablespoon finely chopped fresh rosemary (optional)

    ¼ cup fresh lemon juice

    Stevia (to taste)

Plate all of the vegetables artfully, mixing up the colors, and top with the dressing and the herbs.

the classic daily avocado salad

The simple, savory sweetness of a creamy avocado mixed with stevia and lemon is the ultimate, easy gourmet concoction. Add more avocado to this salad if you'd like it heartier. The more you mix it up, the creamier it gets.

makes 2 to 4 servings

¼ to ½ pound mesclun or baby romaine lettuce

1 ripe avocado, chopped

1 cup grape tomatoes, halved

2 to 3 tablespoons fresh lemon juice

3 to 4 packets stevia

1 tablespoon diced fresh garlic

Sea salt and fresh pepper to taste

2 tablespoons diced sweet onion (optional)

Toss all of the ingredients together in a large salad bowl and serve.

guacamole salad

I cannot get enough of this salad. It's the kind of thing you can eat every night. Since avocados mix beautifully with sweet potatoes, you could round this salad off with a couple of them (topped with a touch of organic butter).

makes 2 to 4 servings

2 Hass avocados, finely chopped

4 ripe Holland tomatoes, diced, or 2 cups grape tomatoes, sliced in half

½ tablespoon minced garlic

1 bunch cilantro, chopped

1 pound baby romaine, mesclun, or regular romaine lettuce, chopped

Juice of 1 lime

1 or 2 stevia packets

Celtic sea salt and freshly ground black pepper to taste

Mix all ingredients together and enjoy.

quick guacamole salad

makes 1 to 2 servings

3 heaping tablespoons guacamole

¼ pound baby romaine lettuce

Place a couple of heaping spoons of guacamole atop a pile of baby romaine lettuce. It's simple and creamy-dreamy!

guacamole

You may use this as a vegetable dip or spread it onto a vegetable sandwich.

makes about 2 cups

3 avocados, chopped

Juice of 2 limes

¼ cup finely chopped red onion

5 plum or vine-ripe tomatoes, chopped (or 1 cup grape tomatoes, sliced in half)

½ cup diced red or yellow peppers

½ bunch fresh cilantro, chopped

1 packet stevia

Celtic sea salt to taste

Mix all the ingredients in a salad bowl.

endive bruschetta

makes about 20 servings

3 Roma tomatoes, chopped

2 cloves garlic, chopped

1 cup packed fresh basil

Celtic sea salt and freshly ground pepper to taste

2 heads endive, separated into leaves

In a mixing bowl combine the tomatoes, garlic, basil, salt, and pepper. Place a heaping tablespoon of the mixture on each endive leaf. This makes a sophisticated, fresh appetizer.

raw goat cheese cabbage sandwich

The closest thing I have found to a raw cheese sandwich!

makes 3 servings

Dijon mustard

3 leaves red or green cabbage

6 thin slices Alta Dena raw cheddar-style goat cheese

Smear a small amount of Dijon mustard on each cabbage leaf and layer two slices of the goat cheese on top. Roll the cabbage leave into a tube and munch.

raw caprese salad

This salad offers all the pleasure of a real Caprese but without the gluey buffalo mozzarella clogging up your cells and pathways.

makes 2 servings

10 thin slices Alta Dena raw cheddar-style goat cheese

2 Holland or plum tomatoes, sliced about ¼-inch thick

10 leaves fresh basil

Drizzle of fresh lemon juice

1 clove garlic, chopped

Celtic sea salt and freshly ground pepper to taste

1 teaspoon minced fresh ginger (optional)

Sprinkle of stevia (optional for those who like a touch of sweetness to offset the
    acidity of the lemon juice)

Layer cheese slices, tomato slices, and basil leaves until each plate has five of each in the colors of the Italian flag. Whisk the lemon juice, garlic, salt, pepper, ginger, and stevia. Spoon dressing on top of the salad.

Raw and Cooked Vegetarian Entrees

simple pasta marinara

makes 4 servings

5 vine-ripe tomatoes

⅓ cup packed fresh basil

⅓ red bell pepper

¼ cup fresh oregano (optional)

1 tablespoon minced fresh ginger

1½ cloves garlic

2 shallots

Juice of ½ lemon

½ cup sun-dried tomatoes

Celtic sea salt and freshly ground pepper to taste

1 large zucchini or spaghetti squash, cut into thirds

Place all the ingredients, except zucchini, in a blender and blend until creamy. Then, one at a time, place each of the zucchini pieces onto a spiralizer and turn until all of the zucchini looks like angel hair pasta. If you do not have a spiralizer, do not cut the zucchini into thirds, rather julienne it finely until it resembles long thin pasta strips. (Alternatively, you may use spaghetti squash.) Pour the tomato sauce over the zucchini.

quickest spaghetti

makes 2 servings

> 2 large zucchinis, sliced into pasta-like strips with a mandolin or a spiralizer
>
> ½ cup Seeds of Change pasta sauce (or Muir Glen, Paesana, or any other natural marinara sauce you like or make)
>
> ½ cup raw Alta Dena goat cheese, grated (optional)

In a small saucepan, heat the pasta sauce well and pour over the zucchini. Toss and top with the goat cheese if desired.

Note: The Seeds of Change and Paesana brands are the best tasting and healthiest bottled sauces I have found (the Muir Glen is very pure but is not as tasty), and they are easy to find in the local health food store. Other organic, high-quality pasta sauces are acceptable too, but look for little to no sugars (never refined sugars), and oil (only olive oil) listed as one of the last ingredients.

sushi to impress

makes 2 to 4 servings

For the Creamy Filling:

1 medium avocado

¼ cup cubed carrots

1 clove minced garlic

1 teaspoon minced fresh ginger

1 tablespoon soy sauce (preferably Nama Shoyu)

2 packets of Nu Naturals stevia or 5 drops liquid stevia

For the Vegetable Filling:

1 medium carrot, julienned

1 medium cucumber, julienned

1 red bell pepper, julienned

Snow pea shoots (if available at your local gourmet market or farm stand)

For the "Sushi Rice":

1 medium parsnip, chopped and pulsed in a food processor until it forms rice-like pieces

6 sheets nori (seaweed)

Blend the ingredients for the cream filling in a food processor until smooth. Place a sheet of nori on a wooden cutting board so that the indented lines on the nori run horizontally. Place a thin layer of the cream filling on the lower third of the nori.

Evenly disperse 2 tablespoons of the sushi rice on top of the cream filling, covering it completely. Place the carrots, the cucumbers, the bell peppers, and the snow pea shoots horizontally on top of the cream filling. Begin to roll the sheet of nori from the bottom, over the vegetables, and then continue rolling until you have created a long tube. Cut the tube into 4 to 6 pieces of equal length. In a small mixing bowl, mix the stevia with the soy sauce or the Nama Shoyu and use this for dipping.

simple raw sushi

makes 8 rolls

     4 sheets nori seaweed

     4 romaine leaves

     1 cup alfalfa sprouts

     1 cucumber, julienned

     1 carrot, shredded or julienned

     1 avocado, sliced (this is optional and can be used when the avocado will combine with the rest of the meal)

Place the nori sheet in front of you. Lay one leaf of romaine lettuce horizontally on top of the nori on the side closest to you. Lay the sprouts, cucumber pieces, and carrot pieces horizontally following the line of the romaine leaf. Carefully roll the nori around the vegetables, pulling it gently toward you as you roll it to make it nice and tight. Then, moisten the end of the nori farthest from you with some water and seal it like an envelope. Slice the roll with a sharp knife down the middle.

Note: You can eat as much of this sushi as you like. It's light and refreshing! Add avocado to make it more filling.

thai delight

makes 2 to 4 servings

3 cups coconut water

½ tablespoon Nama Shoyu soy sauce or tamari

½ teaspoon Celtic sea salt

1 teaspoon sesame oil (optional, just to enhance the taste)

½ tablespoon minced garlic

1 tablespoon minced fresh ginger

1 tablespoon diced lemongrass (optional)

2 red bell peppers, thinly sliced on a mandoline

2 medium carrots, cut into matchstick slices

2 pieces baby bok choy, finely chopped

Meat of 1 or 2 coconuts, sliced into long, thin strips like noodles

In a blender, combine the coconut water, soy sauce, salt, sesame oil, garlic, ginger, and lemon grass. Blend on high until liquefied. Pour mixture over the raw vegetables and coconut strips.

parsnip-carrot-beet bake

makes 2 to 4 servings

2 large parsnips, sliced into thin disks

3 large carrots, sliced into thin disks

1 large beet (or 2 or 3 small ones), sliced into thin disks

1 to 2 packets stevia (as needed for sweetness)

Sea salt and fresh pepper to taste

Preheat oven to 350°F. In a baking dish, layer the parsnips, carrots, and beets. In a small bowl, mix the stevia with the salt and pepper, then pour the mixture evenly over the vegetables. Bake until the veggies become tender, brown, and crispy on the edges (about 25 minutes). Serve on a platter, family-style.

sweet butternut heaven

makes 2 servings

3 cups cubed butternut squash

1 to 2 packets stevia (as needed for sweetness)

2 teaspoons pumpkin pie spice

2 teaspoons organic butter

Sea salt to taste

Preheat oven to 350°F. In a mixing bowl, mix all of the ingredients well and then place them evenly distributed in a baking dish. Bake uncovered for about 35 minutes or until they are soft and brown on the edges.

kombu melt

makes 2 servings

> 3 packages soft Kombu (seaweed) noodles, rinsed
>
> 1 head broccoli, cut into florets
>
> 1 cup shiitake mushrooms, whole or sliced
>
> 1 to 1½ cups Seeds of Change marinara sauce
>
> 4 ounces raw cheddar-style goat cheese, grated (I recommend the Alta Dena brand)

Preheat oven to 250°F. On the stovetop, steam the broccoli in a steamer and heat the pasta sauce in a saucepan. When the broccoli is nearly soft, place the noodles in the steamer (with the broccoli) just long enough to heat them (about 1 minute). The noodles need only be warmed, not cooked, as they are already soft. Place the noodles either in an ovenproof plate or in a baking dish, topped with the broccoli florets, mushrooms, and the heated marinara sauce. Finally, sprinkle with cheese and place the whole dish in the oven with the door ajar for 3 minutes, or until the cheese has melted.

no-fry stir-fry

makes 2 to 4 servings

½ cup vegetable broth (optional; water may be used instead)

1 teaspoon organic butter

1 cup cauliflower florets

1 cup broccoli florets

½ cup shiitake mushrooms, sliced

½ cup julienned carrots

½ cup snow peas

½ cup raw corn, cut off the cob (optional)

1 cup mung bean sprouts

¼ cup fresh cilantro, chopped

¼ cup fresh basil, chopped

1 tablespoon fresh mint (optional), chopped

1 tablespoon garlic, diced

1 tablespoon fresh ginger, diced

1 cup Nama Shoyu

Heat a wok or a skillet on high heat with the water or vegetable broth and the organic butter. In a large mixing bowl, toss all of the vegetables, except the mung bean sprouts and the herbs. Place this mixture in the wok and cook on medium heat for about 5 minutes or until just tender. Plate the heated mixture over the mung bean sprouts and top with the herbs. Enjoy!

Seafood and Other Protein-Based Dishes

beet this flounder!

makes 2 servings

- 2 half-pound flounder or trout filets, rinsed
- 1 cup chopped beets
- 1 clove garlic, diced
- 2 tablespoons fresh-squeezed lemon juice
- 1 teaspoon organic butter, melted
- Sea salt and fresh pepper to taste
- 1 cup raw corn, cut off the cob (do not use frozen corn)
- 2 to 4 sprigs of your favorite herb, such as chives, parsley, or sage (optional)

Preheat oven to 450°F. Place the fish filets in a shallow baking dish, add the beets, then distribute the garlic, lemon juice, butter, and salt and pepper evenly over the whole dish. Bake covered for 25 minutes or until the fish begins to flake. On two separate plates, place ½ cup of the raw corn (you will not be cooking it) and top with the baked fish and beets. Garnish each plate with a sprig or two of your favorite herb to add color and a festive spirit!

simple spiked snapper

makes 2 servings

2 half-pound red snapper filets, rinsed

2 tablespoons fresh-squeezed lemon juice

1 tablespoon organic butter

1 clove garlic, diced

Spike seasoning to taste

Preheat oven to 450°F. Place the fish in a baking dish, add the lemon juice, dab the filets with butter, add the garlic, and sprinkle on the Spike seasoning to taste. Bake covered for approximately 25 minutes or until the fish begins to flake.

has-to-be halibut

makes 2 servings

2 half-pound fresh halibut filets, rinsed

1 teaspoon organic butter

2 tablespoons white wine

1 to 2 packets stevia (as needed for sweetness)

Sea salt and fresh pepper to taste

Preheat oven to 450°F. Place the fish in a baking dish, add the white wine, dab the filets with butter, and add the stevia and the salt and pepper. Bake covered for approximately 25 minutes or until the fish begins to flake and sizzle.

herb-encrusted swordfish

makes 2 servings

    1 teaspoon organic butter, melted

    1 clove garlic, diced

    1 tablespoon finely chopped sage

    1 tablespoon finely chopped rosemary

    1 tablespoon finely chopped chives

    1 tablespoon finely chopped thyme

    Sea salt and fresh pepper to taste

    2 half-pound swordfish filets, rinsed

Preheat oven to 450°F. In a bowl, mix the melted butter with the garlic, herbs, salt, and pepper. Coat the fish filets with the mixture by dipping them into the bowl. Place the fish filets in a baking dish, and top with the remaining butter-garlic-herb mixture. Bake covered for approximately 25 minutes or until the fish is cooked through to taste. (Some people like their swordfish medium rare, while others like it cooked all the way through.)

maple-glazed salmon a la *detox for women*

This is ideal for entertaining. It's so quick and easy to prepare while quite possibly the juiciest, most full-flavored dish your friends have ever enjoyed!

makes 4 servings

1 cup Nama Shoyu soy sauce or tamari

1 clove garlic

1 tablespoon minced fresh ginger

Toasted sesame oil

1 to 2 packets stevia (as needed for sweetness)

4 fresh salmon fillets, well-rinsed

Mix the soy sauce, garlic, ginger, sesame oil, and stevia in a blender. Spread the soy mixture over the fish evenly in a baking dish. Marinate the fish in the refrigerator for 1 to 24 hours. Preheat the oven to 450°F. Bake the fish for about 18 minutes, or until fish flakes easily with a fork.

CLEANSING HAUTE CUISINE COURTESY OF
CHEF MATTHEW BOURDREAU

pan-roasted fluke, raita, and calavanero

makes 4 servings

Fluke

1 teaspoon fennel seeds

1 teaspoon coriander seed

1 teaspoon turmeric powder

¼ teaspoon red pepper flakes

½ stick unsalted butter

Four 6-ounce portions of sushi-quality fluke

Raita

1 cup goat yogurt

2 cucumbers, seeded and grated on cheese grater (large side)

4 mint leaves, finely sliced

1 lemon, juiced

¼ cup chopped parsley

Cavolo Nero Kale

1 stick unsalted butter

2 bunches of cavolo nero kale (Tuscan black—you can find it at some
    specialty shops), chopped coarsely

3 cloves garlic, sliced paper thin

4 shallots, sliced paper thin

1 rosemary stem, whole

¼ cup lemon juice

¾ cup fresh tomato puree

Fine sea salt to taste

Fresh black pepper to taste

First toast the spice mix for fish in oven at 300°F for 10 minutes. Once warm, grind in a mortar and pestle till fine. Reserve.

For the raita, grate cucumber with cheese grater and put into strainer to remove excess water, let sit for 15 minutes. Mix all ingredients together and season. Set aside.

For the cavolo nero, in 1 tablespoon of the butter, saute garlic, shallots, and rosemary until light brown. Add kale in slowly and mix with the remaining butter and the lemon juice to cover kale completely. Let simmer for 6 minutes. Add tomato puree, season, and cook for another 15 minutes.

Sprinkle spice rub and salt on fish while heating sauté pan to medium heat. Add butter to pan and let it sit for 1 minute to gain heat. Add fish to pan and cook for 4 to 6 minutes depending on thickness of fish. Cook the fish on one side the entire time in pan, then flip over the fish at the last second. (You can tell when fish is done when you push the flesh and it does not bounce back.) Place the fish on top of warm cavolo nero then top with raita. Enjoy.

hungry-girl omelet

makes 1 serving

4 free-range eggs

1 cup any vegetable

¼ cup chopped onions

½ cup chopped mushrooms

1 teaspoon butter

Several slices Alta Dena raw cheddar-style goat cheese, or your favorite soft goat cheese

Whisk the eggs in a large bowl. Add the vegetables. Melt the butter in a skillet over medium heat. Add the vegetable mixture and cook until the eggs become semi-firm. Layer the cheese slices onto the omelet. Fold and continue to cook until lightly browned on both sides and the egg is no longer runny. Enjoy with lots of fresh baby greens—any low-starch vegetables will combine perfectly with this dish.

frittata al fresco

makes 1 serving

4 organic eggs

1 teaspoon organic butter

1 to 2 ounces raw goat cheese

¼ cup diced tomatoes

1 tablespoon chopped rosemary or thyme

Preheat oven to 350°F. Whisk the eggs thoroughly in a bowl. Heat the butter in a skillet at high heat and add the eggs, then top with the goat cheese, diced tomatoes, and the herbs. Bake covered in the skillet for 10 minutes or until plump and firm. Serve with garden greens.

Sides and Snacks

chips that won't go to your hips!

makes about 3 cups of chips

- 2 large carrots
- 2 large parsnips
- 1 beet
- 1 zucchini
- 2 tablespoons pure, organic butter
- 1 tablespoon sea salt
- 1 packet of stevia (optional for a sweet and salty flavor)

Using a mandoline, slice all the vegetables into diagonal coin-size slices. Place on a baking sheet. Melt butter and drizzle over veggies. Top veggies with a bit of sea salt. Bake at 400° for 1 hour (or until crispy). Enjoy with a salad at lunch or dinner, dip into guacamole or salsa, or as you like!

guacamole

You can use this as a vegetable dip or spread it onto a vegetable sandwich.

makes about 2 cups

3 avocados, chopped

Juice of 2 limes

¼ cup finely chopped red onion

5 plum or vine-ripe tomatoes, chopped (or 1 cup grape tomatoes, sliced in half)

½ cup diced red or yellow peppers

½ bunch fresh cilantro, chopped

1 packet stevia

Celtic sea salt to taste

Mix all ingredients in a salad bowl.

detox salsa

makes about 2½ cups

8 Holland tomatoes, diced

1 bunch fresh cilantro, chopped

2 cloves garlic, chopped

¼ cup chopped sweet onion

Juice of 1 lime

1 jalapeño pepper, chopped

Blend all ingredients in a large bowl and serve over salad or as a dip for raw veggies.

rocka mole

makes about 2 ½ cups

1 cup Roma or Holland tomatoes, chopped

2 ripe avocados, diced

¼ to ½ cup chopped fresh cilantro

1 tablespoon minced garlic

¼ cup lime juice, fresh-squeezed

1 to 2 packets stevia

Sea salt and fresh ground pepper to taste

½ cup fresh corn, cut off the cob

In a medium bowl, mix all of the ingredients well, until as creamy as desired. Try Rocka Mole in any number of ways: serve it with raw veggies, use it to create a sprouted-grain tortilla wrap, place a dollop on a slice of sprouted-grain toast, or serve it on top of a plate of greens to create a rich avocado salad.

veggie chips and dip

makes 3 cups of vegetable "chips" and 2 ½ cups of dip

1 cup carrots, thinly sliced

1 cup parsnips, thinly sliced

1 cup sweet potato or jicama, thinly sliced (Mexican potato: jicama are hydrating and crunchy like an apple but not sweet)

1 cup Rocka Mole

Artfully arrange each type of "chip" on a plate with the Rocka Mole in the middle for a colorful snack. Grab a chip and dig for Rocka Mole!

don't lose your tacos

These simple tacos are great for kids and parties. Don't worry if you find yourself eating several of them. This is a high-vibration, quick-exit recipe!

makes 2 to 4 servings

1 cup fresh Rocka Mole
4 large leaves cabbage or lettuce

Place a dollop of the Rocka Mole inside the cabbage, or lettuce leaves.

For you Texans out there—go ahead and shake on some Tabasco!

avocado wrap

makes 4 baby wraps

2 tablespoons Dijon mustard
1 medium ripe avocado
1 medium tomato, chopped
¼ cup chopped cilantro
4 large purple or white cabbage leaves

Place all ingredients inside the cabbage leaves, distributing evenly, and enjoy!

part five

DETOX AND EXERCISE

Cleanse First. Build Second.

You will be creating a whole new body with this program. Just as you would never try to rebuild a new house on a weak foundation, you must not try to build a new body before you cleanse the old.

In just a week or two, you will see this eating plan works better than anything you would have tried before, and keeps getting better. It really is possible to look and feel better in your thirties and forties (after having children) than in your teens and twenties. You are not doomed to what you are looking at today. There was a time I never would have believed I could have strong toned arms without regular triceps exercises, or that lean legs were even an option given my body structure. Just sit back and watch how far your body can go and how much more beautiful it can be with nature on your side.

A New Paradigm

The old exercise paradigm simply doesn't serve us. What women tend to discover after years in the gym is that despite all the hours and exertion they devote, they are still dissatisfied with the results. The reality is that exercising in the absence of deep-tissue cleansing is not enough to produce a beautiful, youthful looking body in an adult woman. Its time to throw the old exercise paradigm out the window. (Watch out for falling Stairmasters.)

Keep in mind that the old approach to exercise (gym equipment, machines, etc.) overworks the adrenal glands causing endocrine imbalances that wind up compromising the thyroid gland. Thyroid imbalances are reaching epidemic proportions among adult women due to over stressing the body physically and emotionally. Further, consistent running on concrete (listen up, marathon runners) has detrimental effects on the ovaries, which are also part of the endocrine system. The endocrine glands secrete precious hormones and it's essential that they remain in balance for these hormones to secrete and circulate.

It is an incomparable sensation to be in full command of one's body—to feel one's innate power and be confident in our flexibility, strength, balance, and energy at all times. We should be masters of our body with the skill to leap, push, run fast, reach, and lift at a moment's notice—fighting shape! We can only do this if we are in command and this comes from using and moving the body. We need to understand that the body is meant to be flexible and strong. It is designed to move in an infinite number of ways and combinations. A healthy body is a flexible, strong body.

In the new paradigm, exercise fulfills the following purposes:

1. To maintain the free-flowing expression of Life Force Energy in the body

2. To condition the body by keeping muscles active

3. To obtain and maintain optimum flexibility, which keeps the skin supple, keeps the circulation flowing in the most overlooked places, enables oxygen to reach deep into the tissues, and encourages better breathing

4. To fully posses all the incredible faculties of one's physical body. One needs to feel "in their body" and be aware of their innate power, and be able to use it as needed at any given moment. This is the power of the body.

These goals are a little different from the old-school "gym head" goals, aren't they? When you approach exercise with this refreshingly empowering mentality, exercise becomes much more appealing. It also makes for a much broader definition of what exercise can be and the amount and frequency at which to integrate it.

Stalk Your Own Energy

I recommend an activity I call "stalking your chi flow," which means to take a daily inventory of your energy flow. Watch it and see if it's moving well or if it needs a booster from some form of movement. Then based on what you glean from reading your body's energy signals, determine the best movement for reharmonizing the flow.

Stalking your chi flow starts with an "inner scan" of the body's state. Check to see where things are tight, feel blocked, or where there may be poor skeletal-muscular alignment (a series of rolfing sessions or a good yoga instructor can help you understand desired alignment). Next, check how your energy is flowing. Do you feel filled with life force or a little listless—is it in one area or is it all over? Then, connect all of this with what would most inspire you—jumping on the trampoline (that often wins out for me), going for a short run, dancing around to a particular type of music, breathing and stretching deeply, and so on.

If you've done the mental scan and you're genuinely in flow, agile, strong, and energized, then you may not need to do any deliberate exercise. But if the body needs some fine-tuning that only moving the body in the right way can do, make your selection and incorporate it into your day *as soon as possible* because when the body is in flow, one is inspired. Inspiration is the life force that moves and directs us to greater states of being—better ideas, better communication, and even better relationships.

Get Inspired

The word *inspiration* literally means to have spirit (life force) flowing through the mind and body. You don't want to miss a moment of your day without it or you might make choices that are not for your highest good. We don't exercise to burn calories or so we can eat more, but because we want to feel authentic, powerful Life Force Energy pulsating through us so we can be inspired by our life and our ideas and our relationships.

Why do people seem to keep in shape by working out? Remember that any exercise will help move energy around in the body, which helps mainstream eaters tremendously by improving circulation, conditioning muscles, pushing oxygen deep into the lungs to oxygenate the blood stream and bring about the endorphin rush. Basically, if the average woman ate typically and did not exercise she would really be in trouble. But this does not mean that the common approach to exercise is healthy. It still misses the big picture of how to care for a woman's body.

The Power of Oxygen

Unfortunately, most gyms are enclosed. Pure oxygen is what is needed to oxygenate the body. When you rev up your breathing by moving the body intensely you want to breathe fresh air—not recycled air pumped through filters. This is the big problem by the way with Bikram yoga. The concept of sweating deeply in yoga poses is terrific. Pouring waste through the skin while working on endurance and flexibility is a wonderful idea. However, the pumped hot air that I've seen in Bikram studios is dirty, acidic, and anything but good for the lungs and bloodstream. If you like Bikram, I suggest doing it in the summertime in the fresh, hot, humid air. Exercise should ideally only be taken outside, or with the windows open (cracked in winter is fine).

The *Detox for Women* eating plan allows us to optimally oxygenate the body through the high water/oxygen content of the food itself—and the removal of waste, which allows much more oxygen to flow through the system. So if you do not wish to incorporate exercise into your routine at any point, you will still have terrific results and easy maintenance.

One big concern women have about losing a lot of weight is loose, sagging skin and stretch marks. Have no fear! Cleaning the cells and tissues in this way dramatically improves the outer skin tissue quality. You'll only get tightened and toned even if you have a lot of weight to lose. The new cells will be well-shaped and healthy, making you much more radiant and youthful looking every day! Women are always telling me how surprised they are that their skin doesn't sag after weight loss.

As we will learn on page 166, osteoporosis is best prevented by an alkaline diet, so women have no reason to hit the weight room (unless they really want to for other reasons).

Real Woman: Lisa Rosenbloom,
Marathon Runner and Mother of Four, Los Angeles, CA

My client Lisa Rosenbloom always dreamed of running the Los Angeles Marathon. This was a goal of hers that she simply had to satisfy. I worked with her before she started training (after having her fourth baby), then while she was training. We discussed the stress of marathon running, and decided that despite the fact it was not a way to keep her body young and strong over the long term, it fulfilled a deep goal that she was not willing to compromise. As you'll read in her story, she did indeed complete the Los Angeles Marathon in 2007. She made some very smart choices while training, and now keeps herself in top shape. She still runs on the beach and earth (avoiding the concrete as much as possible), but understands that the lIfestyle of a marathon runner can be damaging if followed for too long. Well done, Lisa!

"In August of 2007 I decided to start training for the Los Angeles marathon, which would take place in March 2008. At the time, I had been following the principles Natalia lays out for about two years. Although I was by no means perfect, at the very least I tried to stick to quick-exit combinations and the green lemonade became a regular part of my diet. I joined a running club; as the training progressed and the mileage increased, our pace leaders stressed the importance of staying hydrated and fueled during our runs. In addition to water, this also meant electrolyte drinks such as Gatorade; and concoctions like "Gu," "Sport Beans," and "Shot Blocks." Having never run long distances before, I was afraid that if I didn't use these products I would "poop out" or "hit the wall" in the middle of a long run. I couldn't help wondering if there was a more natural way to achieve the desired results. I called Natalia and we came up with a homemade "Gatorade" drink consisting of water, raw honey, fresh organic lemon juice, and Himalayan sea salt. Next we needed to figure out something I could eat on a long run that wouldn't be heavy or cause cramps, be easy to digest, and give my body a boost of energy every few miles. Organic Medjool dates stuffed with chlorophyll tablets did the trick! On our 22-mile training run a few weeks before the marathon, it was a hot 84° Fahrenheit outside. While many people from my pace group had to slow down and finish on their own, I felt like I could have kept going as I sprinted the last 100 yards with my pace leaders. On marathon day, I finished my first marathon in a respectable 5 hours and 18 minutes. All I wanted when I crossed the finish line was an ice-cold glass of green lemonade! Three months later, in June 2008, I ran the San Diego Rock and Roll Marathon. I shaved 11 minutes off my time, finishing in 5:07. As long as you remember to eat enough, this way of eating works great even for athletes who engage in a rigorous training program.

Athletes

A cleansing diet is the ideal diet for high-performance, competitive athletes. I work with athletes of all stripes—gymnasts, marathon runners, triathletes, golfers, body builders, surfers, and many others. This program will give you more energy than you ever thought possible. Remember, this is not a vegetarian diet, so there is no concern with losing muscle mass. The only adjustments I make for athletes is that they be sure to eat plentifully and that, depending on how their bodies respond, they may integrate the maintenance program sooner at their discretion.

There are many misnomers circulating about athletes' needs. "Carb-pounding" before a long run, for example, only exhausts the system. Designer protein, soy protein shakes, whey protein, and other protein-based synthetic products are not going to make you a better, quicker, stronger athlete. They will wear down your body quicker, and make you look and feel older sooner. Those packaged sugary items and bars that

---

ON BOUNCING

Rebounding, which is jumping on a mini-trampoline, is the only exercise I do with any real regularity. I started rebounding because it was fun, but I kept rebounding because of the well-being and cosmetic results it provides. A beginner can start out with just five minutes or so, eventually working up to 20 to 30 minutes. The workout can be as gentle or powerful as you want to make it. I find that when I rebound four to five days a week for 30 minutes each, while working the diet, my body easily remains flawlessly lean and toned. I also run for fun now and then, and notice that when I rebound regularly my running cadence is much perkier—almost like I'm running on slightly springy ground. My posture is also much better when I'm rebounding regularly. I notice I hold myself with much more ease and grace.

Rebounding keeps the chi in such great flow that all systems perform to the max. Cellular waste leaves faster, eliminations are stronger, metabolism is quicker, and there is never an iota of water retention. The only times I do not recommend rebounding is during menstruation and pregnancy. Otherwise, I am, as I joke with my kids, "the incredible bouncing mommy!"

are promoted for marathoners, triathletes, and body builders are just dead sugars and indigestible proteins and fats. Replace them with raw honey or dates and chlorophyll tablets. You can mix the honey with water or green juice for easy access while working out. Decreasing the bulk from slow-exit meals and heavy carbs creates abundant Life Force Energy flow. This pure energy that a clean-celled body can tap into gives them an edge in any sport!

I consulted with my friend and national bodybuilding champion Conrad Kines, who has competed and won numerous national bodybuilding competitions, to get another voice on the subject. He emphatically chimed in to say that world-class female athletes (like world-class male athletes) can get all the protein they need from plant-based sources. Just as a horse will manufacture all the protein it needs for its strong musculature from greens, so too will a human. The key is simply to take in enough raw green vegetable juices and salads. Male or female, Kines maintains that live enzymes, plants, oxygen, and a clean system set the foundation for a world-class athlete. He was also quick to point out that, like the male bodybuilders he used to compete with, women athletes eating typical training fare (protein shakes, bars, mainstream food) look haggard and much older than their years. His tip for women: Keep the inorganic sodium intake down for best definition. (Inorganic sodium is sodium from anything other than a non-water-containing plant.) You can learn more from Conrad Kines at freewheatgrass.com.

If you are aiming to build excess muscle, or train for multiple marathons, keep in mind that this is not desirable to the body. Overexertion stresses and overtaxes the adrenal glands, which create a domino effect throughout the endocrine system and, ultimately, all systems. Excessive pressure on the ovaries impacts estrogen production and can lead to abnormalities in and around the ovaries themselves. Overtraining and overbuilding creates a need for excessive intake of food (even if it's the best food) and ultimately stresses the organs, aging the body prematurely.

The Ten Big Excuse Busters

There are a lot of excuses women will use to avoid taking their health and diet seriously. I've identified the ten most notorious excuses below. I hear them from my clients all the time. They are really just stories women tell themselves and each other—and convince themselves are true.

1) I have kids and a busy life

If you are too busy to feed your family right, you are probably taking shortcuts on other things that could harm yourself and your family. If you are so busy because you are doing everything else so carefully (i.e., your home is impeccably vacuumed, your nails are perfectly done, and you are the top contender for garden party president), then you must reconsider your time management and your priorities. Kids and mothers who are living and eating harmoniously function better in school both socially and academically. If there is an unnecessary time drain keeping you from an organic home life, it needs to be deleted from your daily hard drive because nothing could be more important than the health and peace of you and your family. Your nails would certainly benefit from a few months polish-free!

2) I don't live in a community that supports this way of eating/living

Well then maybe it's time to change communities. I'm not kidding. If you live with people who are so closed to change, you might consider how else that community is infringing upon your independent thought and life choices. Most people who feel this way are more intimidated than they need to be. Unless you're living under a rock, you will find that the world has evolved to spotlight detoxification and the green lifestyle. Sure, some in the herd will smirk at your raw salad and challenge you (some with disdainful jealously and others with rapt interest because they secretly want to know more) but that's no reason to hesitate. That's the funny thing about change, it actually requires changing things!

3) It's too expensive

This may be true if you're referring to all those expensive, dense raw food specialty items that are associated with traditional detox, but not with this plan. In actuality, real detox fare that does not include those items is very affordable. For those juicing on a budget, romaine lettuce and carrots make a cheap and delicious combo. Organic produce does not have to be expensive if you buy locally and seasonally. Root vegetables, like baked sweet potatoes, are very affordable and filling, as are millet, quinoa, and buckwheat noodles. You can absolutely keep it cheap, cheerful, and delicious!

4) I have a house full of food. Once I go through it, I'll stop. I hate to waste anything!

Do you know how much time, money, energy, and irreversible damage this kind of mindset does to the body and surrounding environment? That's like saying, "I still have some medication in my medicine cabinet, and when I finish that I'll start drinking vegetable juice for my ailments instead." Or like saying, "I'll start breathing that lovely, fresh oxygen once I run out of this stash of carbon monoxide." When you know better you do better. Find another excuse!

5) I'm always going out to eat

That's great. I'm always going out to eat, too! Restaurants have salads, cooked vegetables, and fish. Next excuse, please.

6) My husband and family will never eat this way. I can't cook two different meals!

If your husband and kids still want burgers, mac 'n cheese, lasagna, or whatever you usually make for them, just make yourself a big salad and let them eat what they usually eat. You could make a giant lunch salad, which will be enough for two meals so you don't have to make it again at dinner. A baked sweet potato takes virtually no effort at all.

The best approach would be to upgrade your family's dinners gradually so that you make a great big raw salad (put out a regular dressing for them if that helps) and fresh fish and vegetables. If they insist on mixing their starches and fleshes, then make a few baked potatoes or some rice or pasta for them. Again, that's not a big effort. Try to find dishes that work for you that they like. Everyone usually likes well-prepared fish, butternut squash or sweet potatoes with butter and sea salt, or pasta made from quinoa or spelt. (Try Vita Spelt brand pastas, which are very good—they even make spelt lasagna noodles.) Don't forget your arsenal of goods that make everything taste great: natural butter, cheddar style raw goat cheese, high-quality marinara sauce, stevia, sea salt, natural spices, and natural ketchup and mustard (Annie's brand is great—kids love it). This is not as big of a problem as you might think. Make plenty for the group, and then just combine accordingly for yourself. Your family's palate will change gradually, making it easier and easier all the time to find dinners that make everyone happy (and make mommy's load lighter, in all aspects)!

7) I'm going on vacation. I'll start when I get back (or I'll start tomorrow or next week).

Vacation is a great time to start something like this. You may not be able to fit the juices in easily unless you are used to making them already, or plan to take frozen vegetable juice, which is certainly an option I would encourage. Otherwise, vacation is a perfect time to start. If you're going away, staying in hotels, eating out, or being otherwise catered to as you would on most vacations, it could not be easier. It's so easy to get fresh salads, avocados, and vegetables for lunch and beautiful salad and fish (or chicken, or even meats in a pinch) for dinner. Have a cheese plate (without the crackers or fruit) and some dark chocolate for dessert, and enjoy wine every night! After all, the whole point of a vacation is to bring oneself back into balance, feel better, explore new things, rest the body, and vacate old ways of doing things.

8) A lot of health issues run in my family. I'm destined to have problems anyway.

Family health problems are a problem because of the way families live and perpetuate their habits by engraining them into the generations that follow. If you've inherited a disease at birth, or before your teens, you have received compromised DNA through your lineage. Your genetic makeup could be weakened by generations of unfit diet-lifestyle, as is the DNA of most Europeans—but there's nothing that could not have been prevented by living according to the knowledge in this book.

Additionally, emotional imbalances manifest in physical ways, so this must also be factored into an illness. This is why we must keep our emotional body detoxed along with our physical body! There's much more to adult illnesses than simply physical genetics. This is one reason some health enthusiasts cannot heal themselves. Healing and detoxification must take place on *all* human levels to ensure dynamic well-being.

9) I need certain foods, like meat, or I need to eat several meals a day or I get hungry/low blood sugar

You "need" them the way a heroin addict needs heroin or like a caffeine junkie needs her cup o' Joe. Yes, your body does need some stimulation because of your diet history, but the high you feel after eating red meat comes from the adrenaline rushing through the panicking animal as it was killed. That should not be confused with the good feeling of properly nourishing your body.

   If you are coming off of the standard diet and have been eating frequently throughout the day because you thought that worked best for you, then naturally you believe that you need to eat frequently. Do this for a while within the parameters of the diet, but once you experience life in a clean-celled body you will see that this "need" was not true for your balanced body but only for your imbalanced body.

10) Let's be realistic, I've had kids and I'm over 35—I'll never look like I did when I was 20 again anyway

Hogwash! Having children does not compromise the potential of the female body for youth, leanness, and longevity in any way. If anything, it only enhances it. The midsection expands and contracts right back to the original size in a clean-celled woman. This excuse totally disempowers women and mothers, and it's all based on living in a false paradigm. Further, the body does not deteriorate because of the number of times one has gone around the sun. It's not one's age but how one cares for oneself and the waste matter that the body either does or does not accumulate as one journeys round and round the sun that creates the appearance of age.

Real Woman: Kris Carr,
Author of *Crazy Sexy Cancer Tips*
and *Crazy Sexy Cancer Survivor*,
Founder of crazysexycancer.com.

February 14, 2003—Happy Valentine's Day, you have cancer. Those words will forever be tattooed on my soul. Thursday, I was an aspiring young actress and photographer living a fabulous (yet broke) life in New York City. By Friday at 2 p.m., *BAM*, I was a cancer patient. To be honest, I thought I just had a hangover, but when my weekly yoga class didn't provide its usual kick-butt cure, a visit to my doctor revealed that my liver was covered with lesions. I had no idea what that meant. Then I got the next blow, the lesions were malignant tumors and unfortunately for me, they had spread to my lungs. The final verdict: an extremely rare sarcoma effecting less than .01 percent of the cancer population. It was totally inoperable with no cure and no definitive treatment. Wow, pass the scotch!

Over the next few months I was scanned constantly to determine how fast the disease was progressing. Luckily, it was determined that the cancer was slow-moving; so in essence, I had the one thing that cancer patients pray for—time. However, since I had no other options my doctor suggested a "watch and wait, learn to live with cancer" approach. I crumbled. Learn to live with cancer? How could I do that without thinking of dying every day?

Clearly I had two choices: wallow in fear or redirect my terror into something positive. Since I equate feeling powerless with suffocation, I decided to focus on what I could control: everything I consumed. And when I say "consume," I mean what I eat, drink, and think. Each is equally important. We can eat an organic plant-based diet, but be so loaded with negativity that our healthy chow choices don't make a dent in our health. Cancer showed me that my life was broken. The fast pace, no time for me, quick-fix life was not only stripping my joy, it was poisoning my body. Oh, and let's not forget the destructive daily bath of self-criticism. Nobody can heal when they become their own worst enemy.

No more. If I couldn't undergo chemo or radiation to get rid of these tumors, I could at least bulletproof my immune system by renovating my life. Enter the full-time healing junkie. I quit my job, sold my apartment, and embarked on my wellness odyssey. The first thing on my list: dump the meat-laden, fake food diet. Pre-cancer, I ate what would keep me slim for my job. Processed power bars, lots of coffee, fat-free this, and take-out that. I was addicted to nonfoods and convenience. I put the crap in, and it was up to my body to figure out what to do with it. Not *my* problem! I was in my twenties—savings accounts, retirement packages, and fiber was boring.

That was the old me. The new me needed help overhauling my diet, so aside from reading every nutrition book I could get my hands on, I went back to school. It wasn't easy because unfortunately there isn't one place where you can get this critical informa- tion. So I had to design a program on my own. The best stop along my journey was at the Hippocrates Health Institute in West Palm Beach, Florida, where I enrolled in their Holistic Health Educator Program. It was there that the pieces of the puzzle came together.

For months, I cut out all animal products and I ate nothing but leafy greens, vegeta- bles, seaweed, sprouted grains, nuts, seeds, and alkaline green juices—including tons of wheatgrass. When I wasn't eating, I was going to yoga, having acupuncture, or getting lymphatic massage. I regularly detoxed through colonics, enemas and implants, infrared saunas, dry brushing, and rebounding. Though I felt awful at first, as the weeks went on I began to feel a sustainable energy and vibrancy that was completely new to me. After a while, I didn't even miss the coffee, alcohol, sugar, white flour, or sushi. One by one, my lifelong symptoms began to fade away. High cholesterol, eczema, allergies, acnes, consti- pation, acid reflux . . . gone. My low blood pressure due to my circulatory disorder and the numbness/cold in my hands and feet improved. How strange, I thought. I have cancer and yet here I am feeling healthier than ever.

Not long after I finished my training at HHI, I met Natalia. Her books helped me refine my practice and offered simple solutions for incorporating my new diet into a real and dynamic life. Thanks to Natalia I was able to take what I had learned in my previous train- ing and make it practical, fun, and sexy! Life is about living, and our food is the ulti- mate energy conduit for our physical, emotional, and spiritual liberation. With Natalia's method, not only can we travel and have a wonderful social life, we can create a deeply compassionate and meaningful life by incorporating her simple principles. Thank you, Lady Rose!

There's no question, cancer changes your life forever. Cancer patients live every day with an indescribable weight on our shoulders. We tiptoe on the razor edge of mortality—

one hand touching the heavens, the other grabbing the earth. Yet so many people who've been through it swear it was the best thing that ever happened to them. Why? Because if we let it, cancer will take us to our zero point and teach us how to live like we mean it.

Today I still have cancer but it is totally stable, not moving. In fact, I no longer call them tumors. Instead they are beauty marks. Will I always have cancer? Not if I have anything to do with it! In my experience, healing is like a centrifugal force. You have to stop something before you can turn it around. But it's important to understand that the only way to stop cancer in its tracks is to be patient and consistent. It may not happen for all, but why not stack the odds in our favor and try? It took many years for the imbalance to occur and it will take time for it to renew. Sadly, so many of us give up when we don't see instant results. My advice: breathe and stay with it. Get back to nature and back to the garden. As one of my gurus told me when I shared my diagnosis, "Congratulations." At the time I thought he was nuts. I now know that my wake-up call was and is a great opportunity.

Please understand that there is no magic pill. Healing, true healing is a remembering. We get out of our way to let the love in. We move, acknowledge, accept, and revolt. We fill our bodies with the alkaline fuel (physical, mental, and spiritual) needed to shake off the darkness. Ultimately, we rescue our minds by changing them. For example, "I can't" becomes "I can." In the end, we may not be cured, but we will be healed.

Some simple tips that have helped me along the way:

Find the right doctors: Before you set out to create your own healing plan and meet your body halfway by changing your diet and lifestyle, it's important to have a trustworthy medical home base. To accomplish that you must become your own advocate, and "hire" the best staff. Do they know the most about your disease? Do they have a good bedside manner, and do they understand that *they* work for *you?* It also helps if your doctor accepts your spiritual beliefs, and is open to discussing alternative or complementary methods of healing that are important to you.

Quiet your mind: *Find a comfortable seat and scan your body for any tension. Make adjustments as necessary. Then focus on one point or your breath (the inhale and exhale are considered one count). If your mind wanders, bring it back to the breath or point and start* *over. Set a kitchen timer to 10 minutes and see if you can slowly work your way up to 30 minutes per day.*

Food is medicine, so get smart about it: Know what you put in your body and monitor how often it comes out! That's right, you are what you eat and what you *don't* poop. Natalia's explanation of food combining not only helps us create a quick-exit strategy for eliminating toxins, it can actually boost our immune system. When our bodies are busy using all their energy for constant digestion there is little time left for repair. Do your homework and don't be afraid or disappointed if your doctor doesn't believe in the power of food as medicine. I wouldn't expect my nutritionist to know how to perform surgery so why should I expect my doctor to be current on all the latest dietary facts? Most if not *all* doctors will admit that they had less than a week of nutritional training in medical school.

Move your body: The body has two circulatory systems: one for blood, the other for lymph, which is a colorless fluid that bathes every cell in the body. The heart circulates the blood. Lymph is circulated by exercise. Many tissues depend on lymph to provide nutrients and carry off wastes. Walking, yoga, or bouncing on a minitrampoline all have great detoxifying effects.

Get enough sleep: Sleep deprivation can have devastating effects on your health. If you don't get enough sleep, your body doesn't have time to repair muscles, boost memory, release hormones, or regulate metabolism. Establish regular sleeping times and avoid caffeine or alcohol. Don't eat for three hours before you go to bed, and sleep in total darkness—light affects your pineal gland's production of melatonin and serotonin, which are the two chemicals that facilitate slumber. Eight hours is best.

Cultivate an attitude of gratitude: Cliché but true. Saying thank you to your body, or to your imbalance or situation, creates a blessed space for healing. As my grandma would say, "don't curse the darkness, light a candle and get busy living."

A Different Perspective on Women's Health

YOUR HEALTH IS *YOUR* RESPONSIBILITY

As you can see from my Ten Big Excuse Busters, I had found that there is nothing more important than taking responsibility for your own health. If you haven't already noticed, we cannot depend on the research studies and the news reports. The research firms are hired by companies with their own private agendas, and they are not testing clean-celled humans. How can we get accurate information on what is true for healthy humans by observing sick ones? The medical community considers someone to be healthy if they are "asymptomatic," or without identifiable illness. Health is not the lack of disease! Health is the presence of undeniable wellness, powerful life force, and undefeatable joy. If this is not the standard at which we set our bar for the human experience, we miss the whole point of what it is to be human and in body. We may as well call it something else like, "sorta-human, no feel so good." Do your testing on me and some of my colleagues, and those who have achieved clean cells, and then give us a "food pyramid" and let's discuss what "normal" and healthy is!

The other thing to be wary of is advertising. Just because something says it will cleanse you, help you lose weight, pile on muscle, melt fat, burn calories, detox you, etc., does not mean it will do any such thing. You cannot take a pill that will melt your fat away. The body just does not work that way, nor will it ever.

You can look great. You can look much younger. You can feel amazing! But not from a product. You need to apply yourself. Starve the yeast and bacteria, eliminate profusely, take in heaps of live enzymes through your vegetable juices and salads, body brush, rebound, and get lots of sleep and it will happen. Don't put your hope in a product or another gimmick. There is no lack of scams (albeit convincing ones at that) ready to take advantage of the consumer who is still holding out hope that something will come along to save her without having to do the work. We can only save ourselves.

You must take the time and make the effort to research and test theories for yourself if you want to be sure you are going to live a truly healthy life, and not be at the mercy of common illnesses and deterioration.

Real Woman: Casey Thomas, 26, Sidney, Australia

"I can't even remember a time when I didn't have eczema. My parents of course took the action they thought would best help me, and that was to take me to the doctor. I was pre-scribed cortisone steroid creams to manage the symptoms. And manage them they did. Quickly. The patches of eczema would disappear with lightning speed, and my skin would again be restored to smoothness. But as the years passed and I hit my teens, the flare-ups seemed to become more and more frequent, and more and more severe. From my early teens, I don't think there was a week that went by when I didn't use the cortisone creams on my skin. As a result, most of my life I appeared to be eczema-free.

"It wasn't until I hit the age of 21 and my personal interest in nutrition and natural health increased (an area I had always been keen on) that I started to question the side effects of the creams, and what they might be doing to my body in the long run. I had been getting sicker more often, for longer, and with worse illnesses. I decided to start researching and found the cream was an immune suppressant. No wonder I was always ill! This started my long, slow journey to try to heal myself with various modalities. Chinese medicine came first, then naturopathy with eliminative diets, allergy testing, anti-candida diets (still cooked foods and heavy on grains), different creams, light therapy—you name it. All of them would help a little, but nothing really worked, and I would eventually give in to the pain-free life the creams could give me, at least on a physical level.

"My skin continued to get worse with a severe flu I had in August 2007, which was the same time I stumbled upon Natalia Rose's work. I realized that the core concept of eating raw and detoxifying made so much sense. Within weeks I was mentally clearer. I wasn't get-ting tired in the afternoons, I felt lighter, and for the first time, I had some sense of spiritual-ity—that there was more than just me. I completely stopped using the steroid creams once and for all, and focused on the end result.

The diet combined with regular colonics, stress management, and addressing the emo-tional link to my eczema means that today I am well on my way to achieving the state of health and glowing skin I desire. My skin has calmed significantly, and although it flares up at times if I vary too greatly from an alkaline diet with less sugar or if I'm stressed, I can now manage it much more easily than ever before. And the best news—I've not touched the steroid creams in over a year! As I continue on this path, the greatest benefits are still revealing themselves to me, that of aligning with my true self and my higher self. That alone makes this whole journey magnificent!"

The biggest women's health issues today have been largely misrepresented. Women need to better understand their own issues so they can make informed choices about prevention and treatment. Below are some of the most common health concerns I encounter with my clients, followed by my admittedly somewhat unorthodox perspective. But these are discoveries that I have found useful. Take personal responsibility and evaluate these new perspectives for yourself! You may find that they help you as well.

Osteoperosis

The common perspective: Osteoporosis results from inadequate calcium intake/absorption. That's what the dairy and supplement industries would like you to think!

A different perspective: It is the acidic Western diet that creates bone loss, not the lack of intake of milk or calcium tablets. Calcium deficiencies that lead to bone loss and ultimately osteoporosis are the result of calcium being leached from the bones by acidic waste matter. The acid waste seeks out alkaline minerals in the body, finds calcium in the bones, and draws it right out—thereby weakening the bone's structure. The same thing happens to the teeth, which are also made of bone.

Up until recently Western women were the only group suffering from bone density loss. Today the "Western diet" has saturated the globe so women everywhere are at risk. Formerly, non-Western women were virtually immune to osteoporosis because of their relatively natural, alkaline, pasteurized-cow-dairy-free diets.

The only approach that will protect a woman and reverse bone loss is reverting to a highly alkaline diet with lots of leafy green vegetable juice, which contains the most highly absorbable form of calcium with magnesium. Any leafy greens will do: romaine, collards, kale, spinach, etc. Carrots are also high in calcium and magnesium, and will make the juice taste even better.

Do not be fooled by supplements or dairy products promising to support bone density. The problem originates from compromising the bone's natural mineral balance and structure due to acidic diet and clogged pathways. It cannot be corrected by patchwork supplementation any more than an iron structure of a building that's been depleted of its iron stores can be corrected by tossing powdered iron on top of it. The bone has to be rebuilt from within, which can only be done with new cells that will spring up in the right environment provided by a clean, alkaline-rich diet.

ALKALINE RESERVE (YOUR REAL IMMUNE SYSTEM)

Your immune system is your ability to fight infection and foreign contaminants. It is not a place in your body that a doctor can point to. Your ability to fight infection is dependent upon your alkaline reserve. Think of it as being a bit like a bank account. If you have a high alkaline reserve, then you can counteract a bit of stress here, lack of sleep there, poor air quality at a weekend conference, a few transatlantic flights. But if your whole life is acidic (acidic food, environment, radiation, inharmonious relationships, etc.) then your alkaline reserve is ransacked, and your body becomes highly acidic. That state, as you now know, is the ideal environment for yeast, bacteria, and the harbinger of general decay. But, if you're drinking your green vegetable juice every day, eating two highly water-containing raw vegetable-based meals a day that are easy on the system, getting enough sleep, and working toward more harmonious life with fewer energy-draining dramas, you will have a huge alkaline reserve. The little stresses of life, the odd compromise at a restaurant or traveling, or a crisis that comes up will not do you in.

So many of these female plagues that we discuss here are due to the body being offended and compromised from every angle—overdrawing the alkaline reserve, and thus leaving your immune system helpless to fight.

One of my clients who works hard in the city in a very competitive field tells me, "Natalia, above all, I just want resilience." Well, your alkaline reserve is your resilience. You can go to all the late-night schmoozing sessions, jet-set all over the world, and yet perform at the highest level with the whole world watching if you do everything else to keep your alkaline reserve high. That means traveling with your frozen vegetable juices packed in a suitcase and "checked" onto the plane (in your luggage, which is still permitted); it means that you body brush every day and jump on your rebounder; it means that you refuse to allow mindless drama to suck out your precious life force. You *do it all* to keep your alkaline reserve as full as you would want that tank of gas in your car or the balance in your bank account to be. Don't let it run out!

Polycystic Ovarian Syndrome (PCOS)

The common perspective: Polycystic Ovarian Syndrome (PCOS) can be corrected by adjusting hormone levels in women.

I get about ten emails a month from women diagnosed with PCOS, which is generally experienced as cyst on the ovaries. It is now the most common female endocrine condition (affecting 5 to 10 percent of women of child-bearing age) and doctors are now linking it to infertility. The medical community is having trouble explaining the root cause of this disorder and mainly blames it on insulin resistance, testosterone, and obesity.

Real Woman: Kristen Conrad, 23

"This is my story, and it is for every woman who's been told that they "can't." I know you have all been told that there are things that you can't do, just as I have. Some of these lines will probably sound familiar: you can't be as healthy as other people; you can't have energy like other people; you can't be as beautiful as other people; you can't be as accomplished as other people; you can't pursue your dreams like other people.

"I have had other people define me for so long. They have told me that I can't be thin—that's just not my "body type." They have told me that I can't be relaxed—that my "personality type" is to be stressed and high-strung. They have told me that I can't pursue my dreams—I need to live a "safe" life and do as everyone else does, going with the typical four-year education plan and getting a normal job. Many people have told me to give up on my dreams. Many people have told me that one person can't change the world. And for a long time I believed all those lies. And since I believed them, they were true.

"When I started incorporating Natalia's principles a little over a year ago, I learned a lot about myself. They didn't just change my physical body; they changed my belief in myself. I proved a lot of people wrong by unveiling a thinner, happier, more vibrant me, the *real* me. And I proved to myself that I am the only one, besides God, who knows who the true me is, everything about me that I am still discovering. Because of that, I am learning to not listen to others' definitions of me anymore. God and I are the only ones who define me. I can do anything I want to do, and my growing and changing dreams are what guide my decisions.

"As for the physical changes I have gone through, I used to be a normal weight of 120, at 5'4".

A different perspective: When the intestine is full due to unfit foods, chronic constipation, and the vicious cycle of putrefaction, the cecum (lower-right part of the colon) and sigmoid (lower-left part of the colon) press into the right and left ovaries respectively. This causes all manner of ovarian trouble.

Also, cysts and tumors develop around an organ as the body's way of preventing poisons from entering the organ. It's no surprise this condition is being linked to infertility; women who are highly constipated and have this type of pressure against their reproductive organs are naturally not going to be very fertile. This is a common sense situation that women need to really pay attention to.

We often try to defy nature to get what we want by ignoring the signposts along the way. If you have been diagnosed with PCOS or been told you are infertile, I highly

I am 23 years old now, and I had been that weight for most of my teenage years, up until a year ago. My weight maintenance approach had been to combine exercise, including weights and running, with calorie counting. I didn't like any of that, but it kept my weight at 120 and I looked better doing those things than when I didn't do them. But I was almost always tired and definitely addicted to sugar, and later, caffeine. I figured I would be at that weight the rest of my life.

"My body changed very quickly when I started the detox. I had more energy, even at night! I dropped to 115 in the first couple weeks. Over the course of the year, I dropped another five pounds, my hair became very shiny, my complexion was glowing, and I felt freed from the impulses that my previous addictions had caused. The energy helped me drive through the night on business trips that my husband and I frequently took. I didn't have to exercise to stay lean, which helped tremendously with my busy lifestyle. I felt great, but I also had a few more pounds I wanted to lose, and I wasn't quite sure how. So I decided to try Natalia's strict anti-candida diet to see if it would work for me. In two weeks I dropped another five pounds, if not more, and gained even more energy.

"There have been a couple months where I have gotten off-track, but I am learning to not condemn myself. It's not about the eating anyway; it's about focus. If my eating is off-track, it signifies to me that my focus in other areas of my life is off-track. Instead of forcing myself to quit eating harmful foods immediately, I spent some time re-evaluating what I really wanted, what my dreams were, and why I wanted to pursue them. The decision to get back on-track became a lot easier once I did that.

"I only have a little over a year of detox living under my belt, so I am excited to discover an even more radiant me as time marches forward!"

recommend taking a year to cleanse your system to the best of your ability, and then try again. Chances are your system will be much more receptive to reproduction, and at the very least you will be in much better condition for anything else you choose to bring into your life.

Menstruation and Menopause

The common perspective: It's normal for women to have uncomfortable menstruation and menopausal experiences.

A different perspective: Periods that are painful, excessively long in duration, give off a pungent odor, or make you unable to function normally are all signs of a toxic woman.

Do you know why women were not invited into the sweat lodges in native Indian tradition? It was not because the men were chauvinistic or wanted to keep their "boys club" segregated. It was because the sweat lodge was developed to provide men with the equivalent effect of the monthly cleansing that women enjoyed from menstruation—the release of the toxicity of a moon-cycle's worth of accumulation from substances that needed to be discarded. The unfertilized egg absorbs the toxicity a woman is exposed to that month. Menstruation releases all that the egg absorbs in a month, explaining why women feel their worst just prior to this release.

When exposed to more poison than natural, the blood will smell bad, increase in abundance and duration, and cause painful cramps. This is not the normal state of menstruation at all. It is another one of the body's warning signs that things just are not right in this woman's world in terms of diet, environment, and emotional stability. Once corrections to the lifestyle are made, periods will become much lighter, shorter, and generally less eventful.

Likewise, the symptoms of menopause are a distinctly Western phenomenon. It's the body's effort to cleanse prior to the next stage of life, and release anything that needs to be "burned off" before the next great threshold is crossed and the initiation to wisdom is made. A clean-celled woman with little physical or emotional "rubbish" to discard will have a relatively uneventful physical transition, and most likely an inspiring emotional and mental one as she moves into this profound stage of leadership.

In terms of caring for the menstruating body, women need to start to pay attention to the links between their birth control and sanitation habits, and their physical imbalances and infertility issues. Regular use of tampons may be convenient in the short term but are a big mistake as they oppose the natural flow of the body.

We never want to jam things into organs—much less those that require a flow in the opposite direction. Tampons fight the flow creating reverse pressure, which, among other things, creates ovarian cysts and probably uterine fibroids. Tampons, even some of the ones at the health food stores, are loaded with chemicals that are highly carcinogenic, and as the chemicals leach into the body, the potential for bladder and cervical cancer and cervical issues skyrocket! The discrepancy between the incidences of female cancers before and after the invention of tampon is dramatic.

Granted, if you need to use one now and then—say for a day at the beach—that won't cause harm. Look for Natren, which is a toxin-free brand. But be attentive to how often you use them!

ESTROGEN RECEPTORS IN ENVIRONMENTAL TOXINS

It's no longer big news that girls are going through puberty younger and men's sperm counts are dropping. There is a crisis in the modern world with environmental toxins that mimic estrogen or disrupt its function. They are called Environmental Estrogen (EEs) and they attach to human estrogen receptors blocking them. They are all around us in the form of chemicals used for personal care products, household cleaners, dry cleaning, plastics, and just about every synthetic you can imagine. They go by names like organochlorines (in plastics, pesticides, and more), Parabens (found in all mainstream personal care products), Phthalates (which are compounds used to make plastic materials more flexible and allow them to be molded and in the radiation and air we breathe), and many more. DDT, noted as the worst offender, is now banned in the United States, but is still widely used in India and China and reaches us through goods shipped from there. We can only control so much of it in our day-to-day exposure, but it's worth being extra vigilant because by doing so we can prevent a lot of damage that these environmental estrogens cause.

There is no question that we must only use organic products that omit these harmful substances, decrease our use of plastics significantly, and maintain healthy blood, lymph, and bowel flow to ensure that these substances have minimal interference with our bodies. The stronger we keep our alkaline reserve (see box on page 167), the better our systems flow, the more vigilant we are, and the more we protect ourselves from the seriously damaging effects of EEs. Again, remember the big picture, as your lifestyle changes, it will have a ripple effect on the lives around you and eventually we can elevate our global community to healthier choices and a better future.

Cancer

The common perspective: Cancer prevention entails regular mammograms after 40 and colonoscopies after 50.

A different perspective: Tumors are the body's way of cleverly keeping poisons out of the organs. Whenever there are growths on the organs it is a sign that the body is working to keep the poisons away, despite the fact that they are close enough to threaten the organs. Once a tumor is filled with poison it becomes malignant. At that point an organ is in danger of becoming as sick as the tumor, which is why it is cut out either fully or in part at this stage (one or both breasts, ovaries, lungs, etc.).

Finding "the cure for cancer" is considered to be the great and noble quest of modern science; there are fundraisers, ribbons, walk/runs, and billions of dollars spent in research. But could the "cure" be in our lifestyles? Could the cause be unfit substances that saturate the body with poisons over time, reaching critical mass in the form of malignant tumors?

If the medical profession advocated a diet-lifestyle from birth that prevented the tissues of the body from absorbing material that could infest human tissue and allow cancers to develop to begin with, there would be no need for a cure because there would be no cancer!

The reason mammograms and colonoscopies are celebrated is because they can detect the build-up of the decades-worth of poisoning before it ravages the organ. But by the time a woman reaches 40, the waste, bacteria, and yeast have permeated the tissues so deeply that precursors to cancer like tumors, cysts, or even cancer itself should not be a surprise at all but an expectation.

Bladder Infections

The common perspective: Bladder infections are due to bacteria getting into the urethra mainly through dehydration, contaminate bathwater, or sexual intercourse.

A different perspective: It's true that bacteria entering the vagina can be the straw that breaks the camel's back resulting in a bladder infection. But a clean, alkaline body can be exposed to all of these things (on the same day) and not wind up with a bladder infection because the true cause of bladder infections is an acidic internal environment where such bacteria can take hold. Create a high alkaline reserve in your body by taking in a diet of at least 80 percent alkaline-forming foods, keep your pathways clear of excess waste matter, and even women most prone to urinary tract infection can avoid ever having another bladder infection. Remember, the body can cope with a little unfavorable bacteria if the alkaline reserve is high. You can think of your alkaline reserve as the power behind your immune system.

Thyroid Imbalances

The common perspective: Thyroid imbalances like hypothyroidism are due to a slowing metabolism.

A different perspective: The thyroid, which is a major gland in the endocrine system, is linked to all the other glands in the endocrine system of which there are seven: the pineal, pituitary, thymus, thyroid, pancreas, gonads (ovaries in women, testes in men), and the adrenal glands. The modern lifestyle wreaks havoc on these powerful but delicate glands that secrete precious hormones in a very precise balance into the blood stream. Modern stress overtaxes the adrenals, which secrete the "fight or flight" hormone adrenalin, beginning the process of sabotaging all the glands. The thyroid naturally gets overworked, becomes enlarged, and is then deemed "underactive"—just as we are when we are overworked for too long and puffy from abuse.

The metabolism, which is often said to slow when the thyroid is low-functioning, is not synonymous with the thyroid at all. In fact there is no such thing as "a metabolism." The metabolism is not a location in the body that a doctor could point to. Instead, metabolism is an event that occurs at the cellular level. Metabolism is the process of breaking down and eliminating foreign substances like food, pollution, etc. When the body is clear of excess waste residue and the cells are clean, metabolism is high-functioning.

Body Odor

The common perspective: Bad breath in the morning is normal; body odor is a human thing—it's natural. Why else would everyone use deodorant?

A different perspective: The stench that comes off the human body is like the waste bin with last week's food sitting in it creating noxious gas. Bacteria run up and down the length of the digestive tract and are the reason that people have bad breath. What you see on the tongue in the morning is a mucus coating from detoxification (fasting from dinner to morning), giving the body a moment to pass some poisons through the tissue while not taking in food. Body odor is also due to the lymph and skin releasing waste.

The armpits are a major lymphatic waste drop zone where millions of bacteria get pushed through as the lymph excretes waste. In this moist environment these little life-forms multiply and grow in size. They should be cleaned out with the alkalinity of soap. Putting chemicals into your major lymph drainage area to stop the flow of perspiration that carries waste out is equal to constipating it. Shoving chemicals into that region creates a double offense.

The lymph becomes overburdened when the body is overrun with waste, and then is further paralyzed by the clogging of the breast and armpit region from chemicals that jam-up the lymph-waste traffic. This traffic jam creates lumps and bumps around the armpits and breasts, which can go from benign to malignant if they collect too much poison for too long (imagine using chemicals to prevent or cover up perspiration since puberty). It is critical to keep that region, as well as the groin region (the other biggest lymphatic hub), free-flowing if we are keep our female organs and glands healthy and secreting ideal amounts of hormones keeping us content and fertile.

Infertility

The common perspective: The infertility epidemic is the result of women waiting longer to have kids.

A different perspective: Reproduction is the privilege of a healthy organism. You don't see infertile soil springing up orchards. Where the soil is fertile, such as in a rainforest, a farmer is not even needed. In infertile ground, the best farmer cannot bring forth life. In the "in-between" soil a good farmer can use his arsenal of know-how, as long as the elements conspire to help with the right amounts of rain and shine to bring forth a harvest, just as someone who makes the effort to clean the system will have a better chance at conception.

There is a reason fertility is greatly on the wane. It's not because women are having children older—that's mostly a big city trend. Young 20- and early 30-somethings are beseeching fertility specialists in droves as well. It is because the modern diet-lifestyle has taken fertile internal terrain and exposed it to enough unnatural substances to initiate a dramatic climate change—rendering an otherwise fertile woman's rainforest a desert. Somewhere in between is where women are finding themselves today and in a couple of generations the desert will be the norm. Those whose lineage has been least compromised by modern living will be the most fertile group, and vice versa.

Infertility is another one of those alarm bells that sound when the body is trying to be heard over the buzzing of conveniences and addictions. The pain of infertility is one of the biggest calls-for-change pains that could be inflicted. The question is, are we going to heed the alarm and see how our ways of living are so obviously not only making us fat, sick, and uncomfortable but showing us our own threat of extinction and make the necessary changes—*or* are we just going to go on partying aboard the *Titanic?*

Men are no more exempt from this phenomenon than women. The male infertility issue can be seen as the literal seed in the agricultural analogy. The seed of course must be rich in life force to generate life. The health of the male is in his sperm, so if his sperm is depleted and lifeless, that is a reflection of his state of health.

By the same logic, erectile dysfunction (ED) is the result of inadequate Life Force Energy. It is inextricably linked to depression, anxiety, circulation, smoking, and general aging in the modern lifestyle. ED reveals a man's inner chi levels. The way Life

Force Energy is circulating in his other organs is the way it will circulate in that organ. It is a direct reflection that could help lead a man to make the effort to start healing internally when he experiences this natural warning sign.

If you take the average man, feed him beer, burgers, donuts, protein powders, sports drinks, and stress and place him behind a desk for a couple of decades or more, his tissues are going to be laden with waste. This waste and stress both diminish his inherent Life Force Energy and they tamper with his endocrine system, where the testes secrete testosterone and produce sperm. Modern living throws the endocrine system out of balance in both men and women.

In short, modern human fertility (and virility) mirrors the state of life-generating potential in our body. If it is a struggle to reproduce, that is because we are too toxic to be reproducing. If we do not face this and correct it, we will only become more unfit to reproduce. We hold the weapon for our own extinction.

SAFE COMMUNITIES OF HAPPINESS AND PEACE

The ultimate purpose of tissue cleansing is not just to get our diets right, or to live longer, or to stay out of doctor's offices and avoid prescription medications. It is to bring an end to the emotional and psychological suffering that is manifested in untoward actions to ourselves, others, and nations. We can make the biggest strides toward healing our world through tissue cleansing. How? The natural state of a clean body is happiness and peace. The corruption of the human body through the consumption of inappropriate food leads the individual to states of pain which can lead to violence, anger, and bitterness.

The poisoning of our bodies leads us to look outside of ourselves for satisfaction—to power, ownership, money, sex, etc. A cleansed body does not have problematic lusts or cravings. Those who do this work start to notice the madness of our group habits, and move toward peace, acceptance, and love. The analogy between the poisoning of our earth—landfills, destruction of the rainforests, overconsumption and wasting of resources, etc.—is a direct reflection of the physical body. As above, so below. If a large enough percentage of the culture engaged in tissue cleansing, great healing would take place on individual and global scales.

Nutritional Supplements

The common perspective: We can correct our body's imbalances with nutritional supplements.

A different perspective: Vitamins, minerals, and "super-foods" are not the answer. They are a waste and a distraction. When malnutrition comes up in blood, hair, or urine analysis it means that the food you've been eating has stuck like glue to your tissues, and the noxious gasses it creates are eating the minerals and vitamins up. All vitamin pushers work off the premise that imbalances can be corrected by replacing substances the body is lacking—implying that health comes from what we put into the body. This is backward, as such an approach treats the symptom instead of the cause, which is great if you've been hurt in an accident, but not if your pain is originating from how you have mistreated your body.

There is only one cause for nutrient deficiencies—the clogging of the body from permeated waste. What this waste does, where it accumulates, and the extent to which it accumulates determines the nature of the imbalance. The poisoning of the tissues from overconsumption of unfit substances simply smothers the healthy, self-regenerating tissue we were born with. When we understand that health is self-regenerating in a clean-celled body we will stop asking the question: "Where do I get my _____ (you can fill in the blank with any of the following: protein, particular vitamin, trace minerals, etc.)?" When poisons are removed through detox, the body can start to regenerate itself without prioritizing of nutrients. An alkalinized, cleansed body never has to worry about the minutiae of nutrients.

Dieting

The common perspective: It's easy to diet back to health and correct weight issues with the leading plans or fad diets.

A different perspective: When someone is eating "normally" (i.e., 3 to 5 meals a day, mixing meats, grain, packaged foods in "normal" quanities) and they are suddenly put on a diet that is restricted calorically, or altered by adding more vegetables and reducing animal proteins and starches, or by reducing or eliminating grain the body has less to deal with and will respond initially in weight loss.

What you must understand is that this effect is temporary, and after the initial few attempts these approaches *stop* working. Why? Because the body is no longer shocked by them and because these diets (other than some of the "cleaner" ones that emphasize non-grain plant foods) barrage the body with dense foods that are very hard to eliminate, so they contribute to the cellular constipation that creates inertia in the body—leading to more weight gain and imbalances.

So while one person is trying a diet for the first time and having some success, another person is exasperated because the same diet that may have worked for them just last year is not working this year.

Detox for Women is not another diet. Properly executed detoxification removes the accumulation that creates the internal constipation and removes the blocks that caused the inertia (slow metabolism). When this is corrected you have a new lease on life—like going back in time. How far can you turn the clock back on your body? Well, the longer you stick with it, the younger you can look and feel. The key is that the accumulation leaves the cells, tissues, and organs.

Colon Cleansing

The common perspective: The colon cleansers with psyllium and herbs work as well or better than enemas/colonics.

A different perspective: This happens to be one of the biggest mistakes detox enthusiasts can make.

Here's an example of a common question I get through my website:

Hi Natalia,

    I was wondering what your opinion is of the "XX cleanse." No need to name one here—there are scores on the market, all promising the same results, and made up of more or less similar ingredients. The promise is that the product is equivalent to getting something like 20 colonics!

My reply,

    Don't do it unless you are doing a daily colonic along with it. Some might get beginner's luck because of how stimulating it is to the intestine, but if you're not one of those the psyllium/bentonite combo will blow you up like a balloon. They absorb 10 times their weight in waste and if that waste doesn't leave the body you wind up poisoning yourself with the same matter again (after feeling so full and sick until it reabsorbs into the tissue). As I've said dozens of times, "If you any of these products worked, don't you think I'd be recommending and selling them?" They are all gimmicks and half-truths. ***There are no short cuts!***

Elimination

The common perspective: We eliminate what we eat. The body can manage the modern diet.

A different perspective: This usually comes as a surprise to people, but fruits and vegetables (and mother's milk for babies) are the only foods human beings were truly meant to eat. The body was designed to pass yesterday's mulch (chewed up fruits and vegetables)—that's all. We can eat other things—nuts, fish grain, etc.—but anything that is not a water-containing fruit or vegetable compromises the ease of digestion and the internal terrain to a certain degree. Obviously there is a hierarchy to the compromises—fresh fish is going to be less of a compromise than, say, a Twinkie. But the fact is only a portion of non-water-containing fruits and vegetables actually manage to find their way out of the intestine. It's true that the body is strong and adaptable when it has lots of chi, but when it is asked to constantly jump through all kinds of hoops at once this privilege is abused, and even our brilliant body gets paralyzed.

When we eat non-water-containing plant foods, we demand our body go to a lot of trouble to move the food through. This is not a big deal if it's done now and then, but when we consume the "normal" diet, the backup of waste eventually fills the intestine. Since the body always tries to keep its centers (pathways, particularly the intestine) clear, the waste then gets pushed into the walls of the intestine, which are multilayered like a sponge. (If you've ever looked at a sponge and seen just how many countless layers are there you'll get an idea of what the intestinal walls are like.) The old matter gets pressed into the intestinal walls to keep the center open for new matter, but eventually those walls become filled with waste (let's not forget three meals a day plus snacks and holidays)—and then where is that matter meant to go? It permeates the walls of the intestine, then spills out into the body at large where it circulates, and then lands somewhere in the organ tissues. Now, as we discussed above, the body works hard to keep this matter out of the vital organs, so at this stage you'll find the matter will go to the skin tissue, causing everything from cellulite to eczema, or you'll see lots of mucosal conditions like bronchitis and asthma. If the diet has been high in starches, you'll see pancreatic issues. If the diet has been excessively rich in cooked proteins and fats, one will likely wind up with liver and gallbladder ailments. A long-term diet that is just generally too rich (cooked fats, cooked proteins, alcohol, starches, sugars, etc.) is a recipe for your classic heart trouble: clogged arteries, heart attack, etc. Alzheimer's disease is a classic example of waste matter permeating the tissues and landing in another part of the body—the brain. Allopathic medicine does not acknowledge that the organism passes waste through the tissues in this holistic way. (Holistic, sometimes called "wholistic," refers to the science of observing the body as a whole organism rather than in parts.) How and when the protein buildup occurs still eludes medical science—but they are clear that this protein buildup is a hallmark of Alzheimer's disease.

One reason the food waste remains in the body is because unfit foods like animal proteins, soy, and man-made packaged foods are acidic and carry a positive ionic charge, whereas the human body is alkaline and negatively charged. When the positively charged acid waste enters the system, it sticks like a magnet to the intestinal walls. This acid waste accumulates and becomes the food for the bacteria and yeast that become the bane of the body's attempt to rebalance itself.

At this point the overzealous self-healer thinks the solution is to eat a diet of raw fruits and vegetables. But this is a big mistake for several reasons.

- When we put only alkaline human food on top of acid waste matter we awaken that waste too quickly. If the body was not meant to pass the cheesesteak you ate in 1982 it's certainly not going to be able to pass it any more easily in 2009! We need to *gently* awaken only little bits of waste at a time so that the body can actually use its growing chi (from good food combinations, body brushing, rebounding, resting from the old diet-lifestyle, etc.) to start removing this waste.

- If we eat fruits (despite how alkalinizing they are) we will only feed the yeast and cause further fermentation, which will exacerbate the yeast and bacteria problem.

- It's simply not sustainable for the average person to eat this way when she is addicted to the kinds of food stimulation that caused this situation to begin with. Therefore *we do not try to remedy this problem by trying to eat only pure food at this point*. Rather, we apply intelligent cleansing as explained throughout this book.

I find it is important to explain how the waste sticks, accumulates, moves through, and nests in the body so that you understand the depth of it *and* the how it can be reversed. This way, every day, week, and month that goes by you'll be able to envision more and more of the blockages leaving your body, which should be great motivation to keep you going strong—gently awakening and releasing the source of your excess weight and ailments.

Please don't forget that going too quickly will only prove problematic. Many people have emailed me telling me that while they read in my previous books not to try to detox too quickly, they did anyway and they were very sorry. They then slowed down the cleanse, their bodies calmed down, and they enjoyed excellent, consistent results. If you are one of those overzealous people who just loves the idea of cleansing as quickly as possible, there is a way to do it, but you must make sure you have access to top-notch bowel cleansing, a la colon hydrotherapy. The frequency of colonics would depend on the level of the diet. The cleaner the diet, the more colonics are needed. The cleansing, alkaline diet awakens the acid waste making it imperative that waste then leave the body. This is the key. If you have access to a good colon therapist and can afford regular colonics, you can quickly watch your ailments leave your body through the waste tube. As the intestine becomes clearer and better able to cope with what it is given, it can start to release what it has been holding in the walls. As the wall too becomes clear, the matter that has settled throughout the body and around the organ tissues can be drawn back through the intestinal tissue and prepare to leave through the bowel. Thus the waste leaves the body in the same way it entered. This is healing.

This is why our work is so exciting: We can turn things around to whatever extent we are able to employ the body's healing help. If we know how to cleanse intelligently and use every outside source we know of (colonics, rebounding, body brushing, sauna sweats, sunbathing, fresh air, rest, etc.) we can turn around just about any condition.

Bigger healing challenges are: (1) those that are so far along they are past the body's ability to have the time to cleanse; (2) those that have come through the lineage and manifested before the age of 12 (which tells us that the illness came through the DNA rather than as a result of self-poisoning through modern diet-lifestyle; and (3) those who have emotionally rooted illnesses that require more than simple tissue-cleansing. Still, this leaves so much that can be healed by intelligent cleansing and offers the best prevention if you find out about it early enough in life.

Nails, Hair, and Skin

The common perspective: Brittle nails and hair are signs of nutrient deficiency. Taking vitamins or cell salts like silica are often suggested.

A different perspective: Brittle nails, hair that doesn't grow well, and skin that lacks a youthful glow are all signs that the Life Force Energy is blocked. Taking vitamins or cell salts to correct this situation is not the holistic or naturopathic response—it's just a theoretical approach that, at best, provides a Band-aid solution. This approach is the same as taking a hair analysis; by seeing what is lacking in the cells of the hair, trying to put that back into the body from an outside source, such as vitamins and mineral supplements. The "pill pushers" of this world have gotten very rich this way.

Here's what you need to know: If your body is lacking in nutrients it is because you have clogged it up such that it cannot receive the electromagnetic current of life that carries life-generating power to cells. Where this is blocked (first in the bowel and then reaching areas throughout the body) the Life Force Energy gets drained, and the body adapts to the energy blockage by making every effort to ensure that the organs get the Life Force Energy that is available. The organs will always come first. Hair, teeth, bones, nails, and a youthful glow—the body can live without. It cannot live without its critical organs. Therefore, when you see your hair, teeth, nails, and skin suffering, your body is trying to tell you that your body has been compromised by your diet-lifestyle, and is struggling to receive adequate life force for everything to flourish. This is the time to make big changes—when the little signs come up and only the nails are suffering, rather than when the body is so clogged that the organs are also becoming starved, which is when the endocrine system starts to go and one winds up with an underactive thyroid and hormonal imbalances.

Imagine your body is like a tree. The roots carry the life force from the earth into your trunk, which houses your vital organs. The branches are your limbs and the leaves are your nails and hair—your finishing touches. When the vital force is strong it will flow up through the trunk and result in flowering leaves revealing brilliant health and beauty. If the vital force is weak or blocked the tree will not flower. A flower is beautiful, but its beauty is not self-made—its beauty comes from the roots, veins that carry the life force of the plant. Of itself, a flower is nothing. This is once again why the drugstore approach to beauty is a fallacy. Beauty is the endpoint of life force.

Eating Disorders

The common perspective: Women and girls with anorexia or bulimia need medical treatment. In severe cases they are sent to specialized centers. Within the walls of these centers, they are educated about what "normal" eating habits are (as if they didn't already know), and are then instructed to model these "good" habits, and in so doing demonstrate that they are okay to function in the world again.

Of course, the women do not actually get better. If they appear to be doing well enough to reenter the world, it's only because they've suppressed their pain more deeply—the pain they express through disordered eating—and once again they have received the clear message that they will not be heard. At a certain point it's easier to numb yourself than to continue to be disappointed.

A different perspective: Many of the common overeating disorders are due in part to food addictions that take over once a woman has become a fully fledged host to yeasts. This tends to happen when we are teens. This is most of what is at play when women go through a loaf of bread or a bag of cookies or chips. These foods feed yeast and the yeast has sent us out to get more food for it. The other part of overeating is connected with the emptiness that women feel and try to fill with food.

But the most rife body image/eating disorder is the one that is so common it appears normal today. The girls I'm referring to may not be outright starving themselves or purging, but they are nonetheless suffering enormously with their bodies and dieting. The average girl is infatuated with having "a good body." It is as common as wearing makeup today, and takes root younger and younger—I've seen it manifesting as early as the second grade!

While it is overlooked as normal for girls to diet all the time now, the fact is that it is all consuming and the majority of girls are actually suffering over the mental focus, time, and energy drain that goes into food and their body. I have yet to encounter a young woman this year who is distress-free with regard to her body.

Speaking as someone who was plagued by this infatuation myself as a teenager, and as someone who has firsthand knowledge about the depth of this insidious focus, I can say without hesitation that it is an epidemic which is a real source of suffering for these girls.

The pretty girls, the thin girls, the smart girls, the girls you wouldn't think even give it a second's thought, who seem impervious to body image insecurities, all have it and think about it, plan around it, and condemn themselves for what they eat and are generally consumed by it around the clock! Most of the time their parents know and ignore it—either because they have the same issues themselves or they have been projecting the importance of being slim onto their daughters, and see nothing wrong with it.

Some of my clients have reported that when they were practicing the most severe forms of their eating disorders they received the most effusive acceptance from their family and peers. Imagine how confusing that is!

It's high time the reality is unveiled. The fact is that most are suffering and the only way to truly remedy the problem is to face up to the fact that the social norms around food go against natural law. If you want a "good body" you need to eat according to natural law.

I have held the hands of numerous anorexics and bulimics across the threshold back to balance using the dietary guidelines in my books; along with a thorough dredging (and releasing) of (1) the true origin of their anger; (2) what they truly long to express that they feel they cannot; and (3) their depth of social programming so they can be free to be more authentic and have fewer and fewer reasons to use their throat as a weapon of exploding emotion—instead of a pathway for honestly and freely expressing themselves and serving themselves foods rich in life force and flavor. They need truth served up in hearty quantities. Food intake should consist of fresh vegetable juice and raw salads with avocado and baked roots so they can discover the liberating truth: food can be nourishing and satisfying, and can keep them looking beautiful and lean.

In my experience, the most effective way to eliminate an eating disorder is to give the woman the following tools for breaking free of the big-picture belief system that caused them.

She needs to know that she does not have to conform to "normal" ways of eating to be healthy, strong, or socially acceptable.

She needs to lose her fears around eating by seeing for herself that she can get pleasure and satisfaction from food while feeling light in her body and loving the way she looks. Note: This is usually the most important factor and the one that makes all women with all levels of food issues sigh with relief and liberated delight!

She needs to have a safe place to dredge up what it is she really wants to say, and say it again and again until she feels heard by someone who can listen (and is not an inanimate object with flushing capabilities) with complete receptivity.

She needs to be shown that the adults in her life were just repeating what they knew. Just as she couldn't be angry at a first grader for not being able to do advanced calculus, it is easier to forgive a parent or other authority if it is understood that they were simply not aware that the way they were living and what they engrained in her was misguided.

Finally, she must see there are many who do not subscribe to old ways of thinking, living and relating. With my young clients (late-teens, early-twenties), I do my best to link them up with each other. They take to each other immediately, and usually wind up becoming great friends who can understand and support each other. It's really important that they don't feel alone—it would be a real pity since they are not alone!

More of these young people who have chosen to walk away from the painful choices that made them turn to eating disorders, drugs, and alcohol and toward a more enlightened approach need to find each other and live out their highest ideals with each other's support and companionship. As this is encouraged and facilitated by savvy, caring grown-ups, the suffering will diminish.

Cleansing the Macrocosmic Cells

To see a World in a Grain of Sand
And a Heaven in a Wild Flower
Hold Infinity in the palm of your hand
And Eternity in an hour.

WILLIAM BLAKE, *AUGURIES OF INNOCENCE*, 1794

There is a universal natural law called The Law of Correspondences. The Law of Correspondences is a fancy way of saying that what is true for the smallest things is also true for larger things. Another way this law is often presented is, "As above so below; as below so above. As within so without; as without so within." What this means is that what is true at the cellular level is also true at much larger levels of life—our solar system and universe. Life is expressed with extraordinary similarity on the most microcosmic and macrocosmic levels.

Your life is filled with microcosmic and macrocosmic relationships that you may not be aware of. The moment the correspondences between the health of your cells and the health of your human "cell" and community "cell" dawn on you, you will immediately see how cellular cleaning on a physical level directly affects all the "cells" and "tissues" of your life. You can take the concept of the cell health and see how all the areas of your life (emotions, relationships, home life, work life, etc.) correspond with each other.

Your Life as a "Cell"

Let's take your life as "the cell" and have a look at how clean and functional it is. On a physical level, there's your environment. Is your home organized or filled with disorganized "waste" (pack rat stuff, unnecessary items, and so on)? Is it mostly natural, or "unfit" for consumption (wall-to-wall carpeting, synthetic materials, radiation from excess wireless exposure, microwaves)? Is it rife with acidic emotions and relationship dramas (family fighting, resentment toward those in your "organism," unconstructive pressures, anger, repressed pain)?

We need to look at our environment in the same way we would look at our cells in our body. Remember in the beginning of the book when I said you could look at your face and see the state of your insides? At this level of correspondence you can look at your heart and feel the true state of your life.

If you have children, they are as close to your physical heart manifested in form as you will come, so you could also look at them—if you can do so without filters, blinders, or rose-colored glasses. They will reflect you (and your spouse, of course) and show you things about yourself that you will truly benefit from seeing.

In this same way, if we pull way, way out, we can see the cleanliness of "the cell" of our world by looking at our world's plants, animals, orphans, and dependent adults—the elderly, the psychologically unwell, the handicapped. Those who are dependent will almost always reveal the inner nature of that which has dominion over them. In this case, these things mirror to us the corporate values of our human race.

A clean-celled individual will function harmoniously, contributing to communities of, ideally, clean-celled individuals who will likewise have a harmonious effect on the larger global community manifesting in a peaceful, healthy, love-generating planet. This is the goal and when we look at the Law of Correspondences we can see how to heal the world at the macrocosmic level by taking microcosmic steps.

In Closing

Everything you need to know about the care of a woman's body you can know by observing a garden. Where the life-generating elements are present (pure water, plenty of sunshine, nutritionally balanced, healthy soil, fresh air, and good seeds) it will be beautiful—like a rainforest of colors, plant life, oxygen, rich, intoxicating air. If that soil is imbalanced, pests will come. If the water is acidic or carries poisons, if there is inadequate sunlight, trash thrown about the garden, and lifeless air circulating, the garden will be unhealthy, unappealing, and most certainly infertile. Caring for the female body is not a mystery. It is as clear and available for the understanding as how to grow a garden.

When the body of a woman is tilled correctly there is no makeup that could compare to her skin, hair, and eyes, and no garment cut so finely as her own irresistible curves. Left in the hands of a good gardener, she would be attired in the greatest splendor.

If we apply the Law of Correspondences to the macrocosmic network of life we can see how our global family depends on the choices we make as individuals, which determine the state of our cells, tissues, and organs. If we can overcome the harmful legions, we can overcome on all levels; if we are overcome by them, we will be overcome in all ways.

We are responsible for what happens next. Will we choose the path of least resistance and give into our addictions and programming around acidic choices—or redirect ourselves toward healing choices that will enable good, alkaline energy to unquestionably maintain the power and peace of our global body?

Women hold enormous power in determining how the global garden will grow. If we adopt the truths of self-care in our own lives, and teach our receptive family members and friends in gentle respectful ways, we can effectively secure the balance of power and healing back in our bodies and throughout the planet as a whole.

By understanding how the whole thing works on the microcosmic and macrocosmic levels and integrating it according to our sphere of influence, we can turn a losing match into a victorious one! First we set ourselves right, then we can take a look at our families and larger communities.

Women are the healers, the nurturers, the leaders. American and Western women are free to use what they know to choose any direction to pursue anything they want. We are free. The question stands before you: Are you going to exercise that freedom? Are you going to tap your own natural powers of healing? If you do, I can guarantee your life and all life will take a quantum leap forward in health, beauty, and joy.

Acknowledgments

I would first like to thank the women who shared their stories in this book. Sarah Appleton, Susie Castillo, Casey Thomas, Jennifer Gonzalez, Kristen Conrad, Lisa Rosenbloom, and Kris Carr: You are all beautiful, inspirational, brilliant women and I greatly admire all of you for what you bring to our group consciousness every day. You make the sisterhood great! Thank you for being courageous and bold and sharing your stories.

To Britanie King, my wonderful intern, thank you for all the enthusiasm you brought to this project. You were a godsend!

A very special thank you to Caroline Sutton, my editor at HarperCollins, for her keen eye, dedication, and care—as well as to Mary Ellen O'Neill at HarperCollins for believing in me and this critically important topic and shepherding it through.

A standing ovation goes to my beloved teacher and friend Gil Jacobs, without whom I never would have made my way through the maze of alternative healing. Gil, you have been a beacon of light, showing me every next turn and preventing all wrong turns! My gratitude to you is immeasurable.

I am so thankful to my brother, Roman Barrett, who stepped in at the eleventh hour to shoot the cover photo for this book. Also, very special recognition needs to be given to my assistant-cum-protégée-cum-business manager, Ana Ladd-Griffen, who has helped me manage house, children, clients, and the booming Detox the World community. To that end, I would like to thank web developers Tim and George Roberts for their immense creativity and dedication. I would also like to extend my deepest gratitude to J.R.—thanks for the use of your kitchen and so much more!

My children Thandi and Tommy serve up my daily inspiration to understand as much as I can about the body and our life's purpose. In fact, it was in my role as mother that I realized how critical living in harmony with natural laws was for positive human evolution and the protection of our precious humanity.

To my husband Lawrence: Thank you for supporting me every step of the way and giving me the space to explore unconventional ideas. Thank you for sharing your life with me (and not sending food back to the kitchen). I love you.

To my readers, I thank you for entrusting me with your bodies and hopes. I care deeply for you and the healing of our human family. It is my sincerest wish that you benefit tremendously from this information.

With love in union,
Natalia Rose
New York City, June 21, 2008
For more information on Natalia Rose
and her work, visit DetoxTheWorld.com.

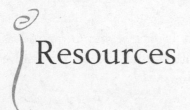

Resources

THE INTERNATIONAL COLON THERAPY DIRECTORY

UNITED STATES OF AMERICA

ARIZONA

Intestinal Health Institute
East Fifth Street west of Swan and east of Columbus roads,
Tucson, AZ
Therapist: Sheila Shea
Phone: 520-325-9686
Email: sheila@intestinalhealthinstitute.com

Ancient Waters Colon Therapy
Oracle and El Conquistidor Way
Tucson, AZ 85737
Therapist: Ann Schnell
Phone: 520 575-5812
Email: ancientwaters@hotmail.com
Website: www.ancientwaters.info

CALIFORNIA

Healing Waters Gravity Flow
26 East Sola Street, Santa Barbara, CA 93102
Therapist: Suzie Sebastian
Phone: 805-453-2942

Holistically In Tune
1024 Pico Blvd #8, Santa Monica, CA 90405
Therapist: Fatima Lowe-Williams, I-ACT Certified
Phone: 213-453-8926
Email: holistic1@yahoo.com
Website: www.holisticallyintune.com

Inner Light
San Francisco Bay Area
Phone: 415-690-0356
Email: elena@innerlightcleansing.com
Website: www.innerlightcleansing.com
2633 Windmill View Rd., San Diego, CA 92020
Millan Chessman (I-ACT Instructor Certified Therapist)
Phone: 619-562-5446 or 800-311-8222

Cindy Paiva
San Francisco Bay Area
Phone: 510-409-3662
Email: gravitycolonics@gmail.com

CONNECTICUT

Xell Calderer
Internal Hygiene and Wellness
Woods Gravity Method
Phone:203-524-2888
Email: internalhygiene@gmail.com
Website: www.internal-hygiene.com

GEORGIA

Midtown Atlanta Wellness Center
117 5th Street, NE, Suite 1, Atlanta, GA 30308
Therapist: Tanya Molinelli (I-ACT Advanced Certified Therapist
and LIBBE Certified Therapist)
Phone: 404-347-9444
Fax: 404-347-9443
Email: info@midtownatlantawellness.com
Website: www.midtownatlantawellness.com
FDA equipment—LIBBE* (disposable tubes)

*Note that both gravity and pressure modes are offered so be sure to ask
for the former.*

The Star Wellness Center
Sandy Springs Location:
275 Carpenter Drive, Suite 202, Atlanta, GA 30328
Therapist: Mary Cote (I-ACT certified therapist)

Virginia Highlands Location:
1097 Briarcliff Place NE, Atlanta, GA 30306
Phone: 404-497-9268 (for both locations) and Fax: 404-876-3820
Email: joseph@starwellnesscenter.com
Website: www.starwellnesscenter.com

ILLINOIS

The Chicago Wellness Center
1900 W. Addison
Chicago, IL 60613
Phone: 773-935-9147

MASSACHUSETTS

The Natural Path Alternative
214 Market Street, Brighton, MA 02135
Phone: 617-787-5040 and Fax: 617-787-5834
Email: colonics@earthlink.net
Website: www.healthycleansing.com

Hampshire Colon Hydrotherapy
25 Holyoke Street
Easthampton, MA 01027
Phone: 413-527-8332
Linda Whitford; Certified Colon Hydrotherapist

NEW MEXICO

Ann Marie Roth, NTS, LMT #5350
Vitality Works
126 Quincy St NE
Albuquerque, NM 87108
Phone: 505-280-3615
Website: www.vitalityworksnm.com

NORTH CAROLINA

Wellville Massage & Hydrotherapy
2101 Chapel Hill Road
Durham, NC
Therapist: Kim Dupre
Phone: 919-730-4542
Email: wellville1111@yahoo.com

NEW JERSEY

A Touch of Warmth
Main Street, Edison, NJ 08840
Therapist: Linda Durren
Phone: 732-738-3800
Email: linda@colonicsinnj.com or touchofwarmth@aol.com
Website: colonicsinnj.com

NEW MEXICO

Janetta Penderson
Las Cruces, NM
Phone: 575-621-3195

NEW YORK

Axis—A New Space by Gil Jacobs
528 E. 5th Street #1B, New York, NY 10009
Phone: 917-435-9196
Website: www.lytnyc.com

*Gil Jacobs
528 E. 5th Street, New York, NY 10009
Therapist: Gil Jacobs
Phone: 212-254-5279

LYT
5th Avenue @ 34th Street
Phone: 212-696-1800
Website: www.lytnyc.com
Open 7 days

Ask for Cyndie, Joyce, Armando, Mavon, or Michelle who are all fabulous, certified Woods Gravity practioners, and trained by Gil Jacobs himself!

*Hands down, Gil Jacobs is the best and most knowledgeable colon therapist (and health educator) in the world. If you are close to NYC, it would be a shame to miss out on experiencing his treatments and his insights!

Ascend Colonics (In Queens!)
Therapist: Seth Block
Phone: 347-558-9845
Email: information@ascendcolonics.com

OREGON

Chakra 17 West
Phone: 503-493-9656
Website: chakra17.com

Chakra 17 West is easily the best colon hydrotherpay practice on the west coast. It's founder, Wendy Jones, was part of the orignial team of Gil Jacob's trained therapists. Wendy is exceptionally knowledgeable about all aspects of the cleansing lifestyle. Alec Steury and Kristen Andolino are also part of her expert group and get rave reviews!

TEXAS

Balanced Approach Holistic Health
Oakwood Tower, 3626 N. Hall St. Suite 500, Dallas, TX 75219
Therapist: Pamela Karon (I-ACT Instructor Certified Therapist)
Phone: 214-520-0216
Website: www.balancedapproach.com
Gravity-centered & both open and closed system

VIRGINIA

Healthy Muse–Athanor Hydrotherapy Center
487-A Carlise Drive, Herndon, VA 20170 (Washington, DC
Metropolitan Area)
Therapists: Caroline Elizabeth Alexander (I-ACT Certified
Instructor and National Board Certified), Brenda White and Megan
Scango (I-ACT Foundation Certified Therapists)
Phone: 703-953-3323
Email: athanorhydrotherapy@comcast.net
Website: www.healthymuse.com
FDA Equipment (Angel of Water open system—a gravity-fed
system)
Rectal nozzles are disposable.
Both open and closed systems are gravity-fed system.

WASHINGTON STATE

INNERGY
345 Knechtel Way, N.E.
Suite 202
Bainbridge Island, WA 98110
Therapist: Marie Pence
Phone: 206-842-4505

*Marie has 35 years of colon hydrotherapy experience with the gravity
method and was trained by Dr. Bernard Jensen in the early 1970s.
She also served on staff at the original Hippocrates Health Institute in
Boston in the mid 1970s and worked alongside Dr. Ann Wigmore for three
years. Many of her clients fly in from elsewhere just to be treated by Marie!
Her office is walking distance off the ferry from Seattle.*

CANADA

BRITISH COLUMBIA

Vestta Whole Health Centre
1138 Richards Street, Vancouver, BC V6B 3E6
Therapist: Lizette Kilpatrick
Phone: 604-731-3571 and Toll free: 1.866.3VESTTA
Website: www.vesttawholehealth.com
Gravity-centered & closed system

ONTARIO

D'Avigon Digestive Health Center
113 Danforth Avenue (at Broadview), Toronto, ON M4K 1N2
Therapist: Louise Comtois
Phone: 416-465-1222
Email: contactus@digestivehealthcentre.com
Website: www.digestivehealthcentre.com

ENGLAND

Balance
The Courtyard, 250 Kings Road, Chelsea SW3 5UE
Phone: 020 7565 0333
Email: enquiries@balancetheclinic.com
Balance gets rave reviews from my friends and clients in the UK!

Brackenbury Natural Health Clinic
30 Brackenbury Road, London W6 0BA
Phone: 020 8741 9264
Gravity-centered & closed system

Chelsea Healing Rooms
402 Kings Road (under Chelsea Health Store), London SW10 0LJ
Phone: 020 7352 4774
Gravity-centered & closed system

SOUTH AFRICA

**Lawson's Wellness Center (a retreat)
Plettenberg Bay
Therapist: Kate Forbes
Phone: 011-27-84-532-7838 or 011-27-84-980-5434
Email: kate@sustainablehealth.co.za

Kate Forbes is top-notch. I highly recommend her if you are so lucky to find yourself in this exquisite corner of the world!

The Colon Health Centre
Cape Town
29 Wrensch Rd
Observatory
Cape Town 7925
Therapist: Rosabla
Phone: 2721-448-5562

This is where I go when I'm in Cape Town. Rosabla is a radiant, expert colon therapist. I absolutely adore her!

Stellenbosh
The HYDRO
High Rustenberg Estate
Phone: 27 21 809 3800

The HYDRO is out of another place in time. It is a must visit for anyone into health in the area. Nurses referred to as "Sisters" administer the colonics. They have wonderful services across the board and I just find the entire retreat enchanting.

Note: The LIBBE system stands for Lower Intestine Bottom Bowel Evacuation System. It is an FDA Registered (Class II) medical device.

Index

ALSO BY NATALIA ROSE

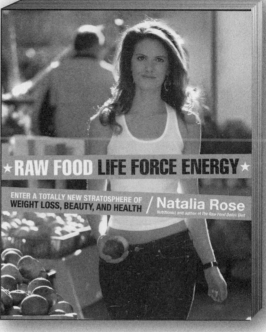

ISBN 978-0-06-083437-1 (paperback)

ISBN 978-0-06-134465-7 (paperback)

"The true 'anti-fad' diet . . . There's no deprivation with this regimen—just satisfaction, with slimming results."
—*Hamptons* magazine

"An easy, ultra-effective diet you're gonna love!"
—*Woman's World*

"In clear, inspiring language, Rose explains how your body responds to various foods and food combinations. This book helps you put the science of enzymes to work for better health."
—*Total Health*

Looking for a whole new approach to weight loss, health, and beauty without necessarily going all-raw or strictly vegetarian? Natalia Rose offers a new vision of how to honor and revitalize our bodies and become powerfully attractive inside and out. *Raw Food Life Force Energy* shows us how to break out of our destructive, energy-draining patterns of poor eating, unsuccessful dieting, and stressful living to lift ourselves to a whole new stratosphere of well-being.

WM
WILLIAM MORROW
An Imprint of HarperCollins*Publishers*

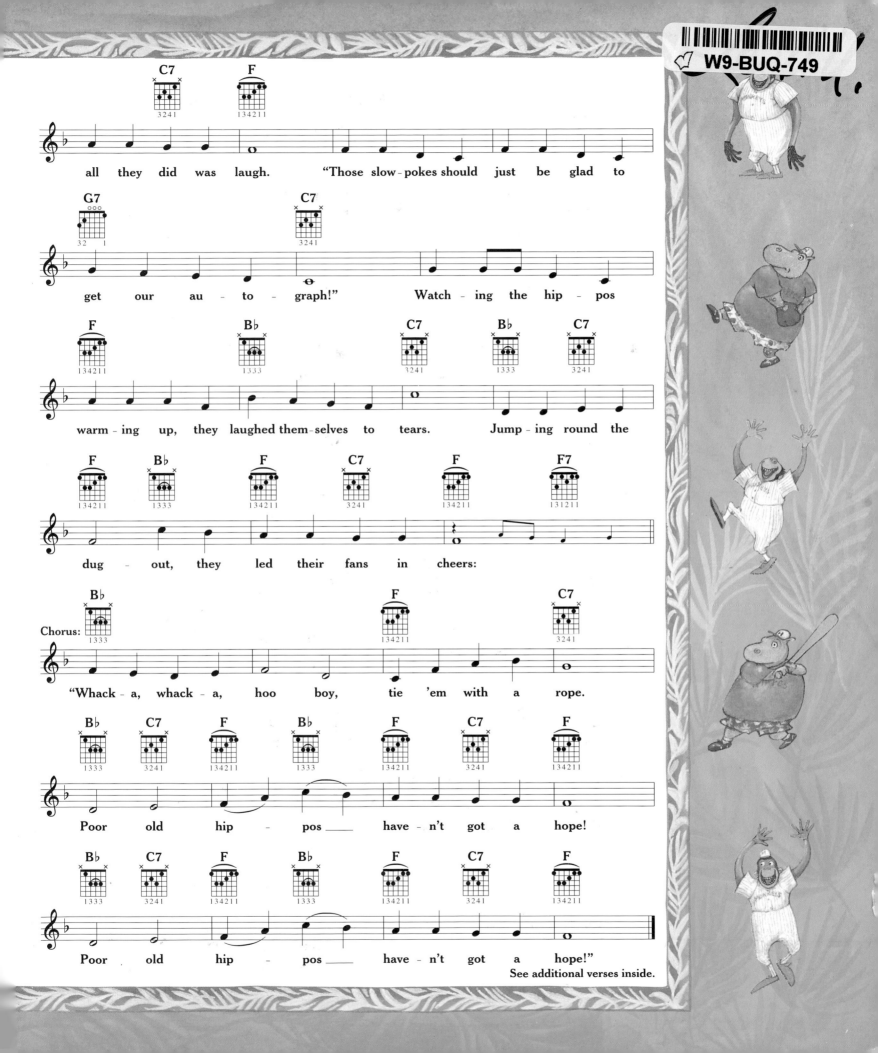

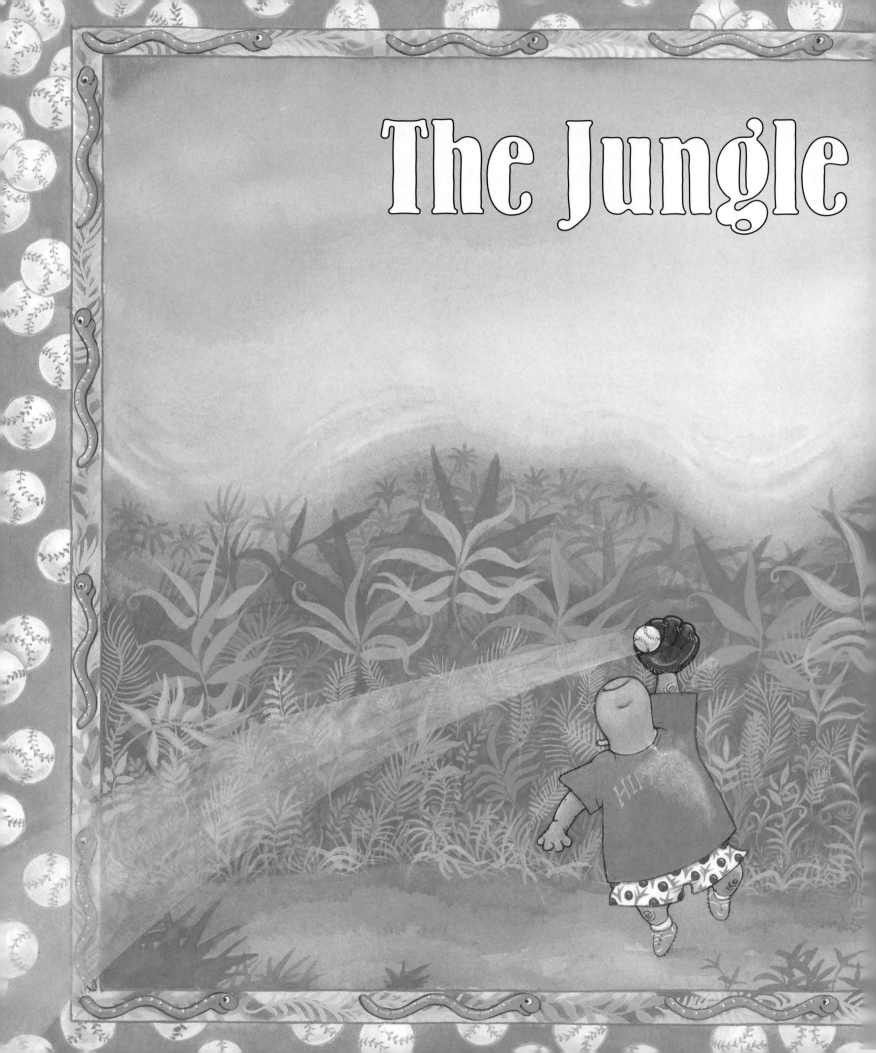

The Jungle

Baseball Game

BY
Tom Paxton

ILLUSTRATED BY
Karen Lee Schmidt

MORROW JUNIOR BOOKS • New York

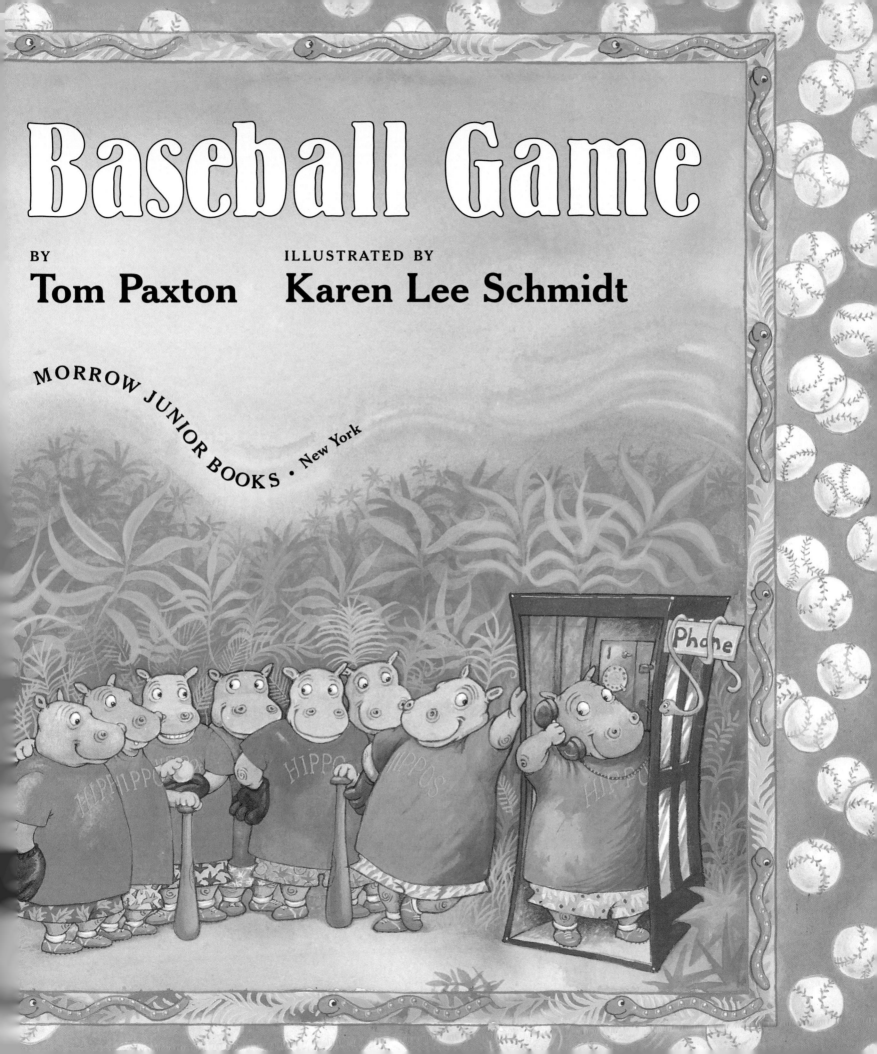

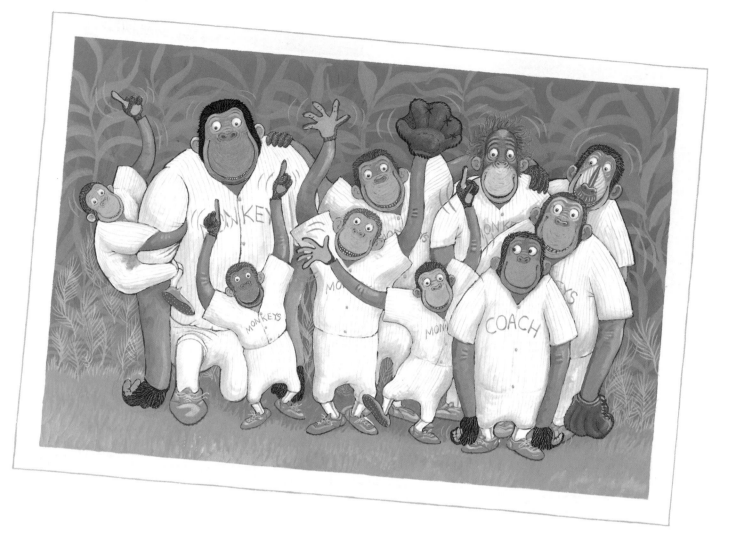

Watercolor and gouache were used for the full-color illustrations.
The text type is 20-point Cheltenham.

Published by Morrow Junior Books, a division of William Morrow and Company, Inc.,
1350 Avenue of the Americas, New York, NY 10019.

Printed in Singapore at Tien Wah Press.

1 2 3 4 5 6 7 8 9 10

Library of Congress Cataloging-in-Publication Data
Paxton, Tom.
The jungle baseball game/by Tom Paxton; illustrated by Karen Lee Schmidt.
p. cm.
Summary: The jungle animals enjoy a rousing game of baseball.
ISBN 0-688-13979-5 (trade)—ISBN 0-688-13980-9 (library)
[1. Jungle animals—Fiction.   2. Baseball—Fiction.]   I. Schmidt, Karen, ill.
II. Title.   PZ8.3.P2738Ju 1999   [E]—dc21   97-6459   CIP   AC

To Petey and Daisy Landi,
in honor of their grandfather and my friend
Peter Dohanos
—T.P.

To my aunt Clara H. Brown,
for friendship and early morning waffles
—K.L.S.

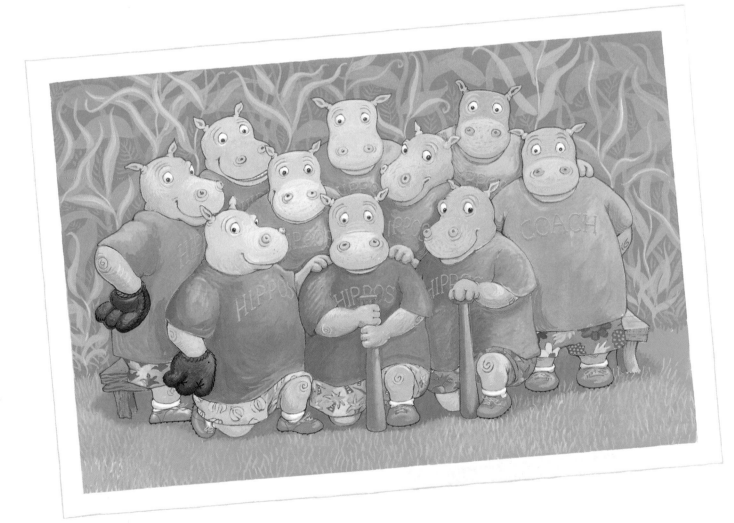

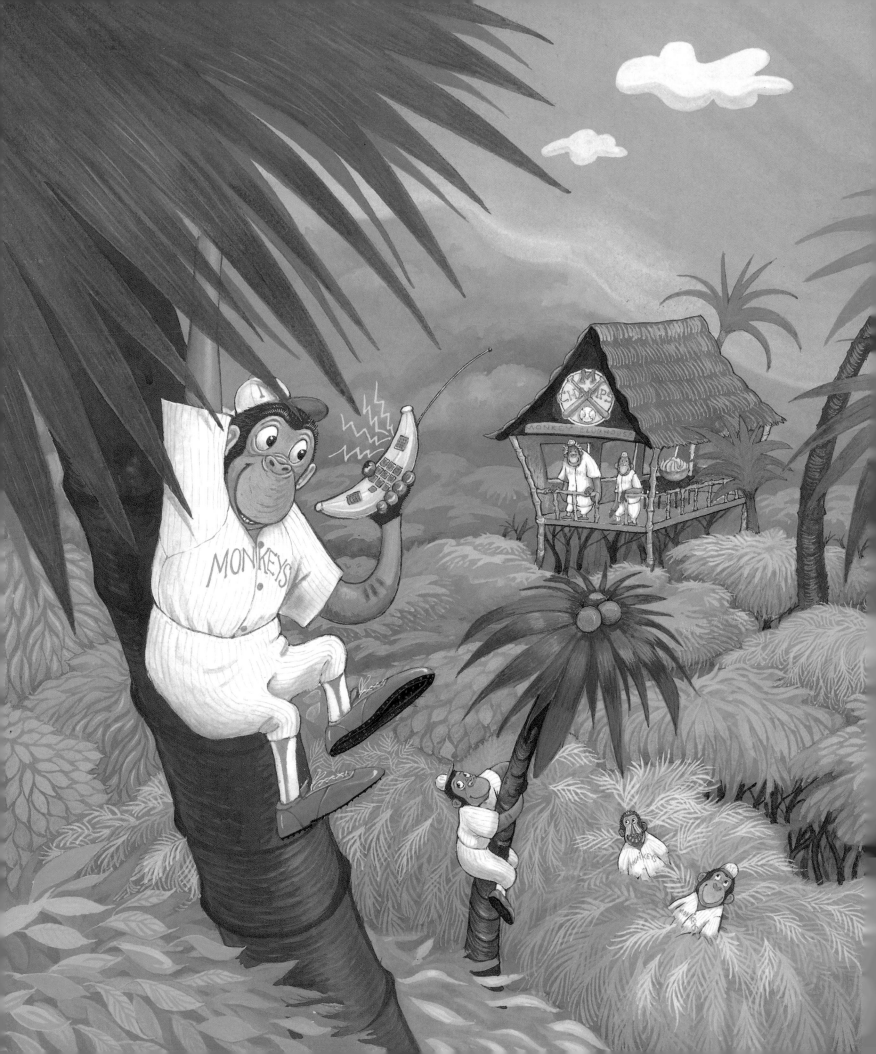

Rang-alang-lang, the telephone rang,
Way up in the coconut tree.
Mister Monkey ran to answer—
"Someone's calling me."
Mister Hippo, on the line,
Yelled, "Am I getting through?
Get your monkey baseball team—
We want to play ball with you."

When the monkeys saw the hippos,
All they did was laugh.
"Those slowpokes should just be glad
To get our autograph!"

Watching the hippos warming up,
They laughed themselves to tears.
Jumping round the dugout,
They led their fans in cheers:

"Whacka, whacka, hoo boy,
Tie 'em with a rope.

Poor old hippos
Haven't got a hope!"

A chimpanzee played out in left;
A baboon stood in right.
The orangutan on the pitcher's mound
Was a most impressive sight.

Little monkeys in the field
Were the quickest ones of all.
Far as the hippos hit the pitch,
Those monkeys caught the ball.

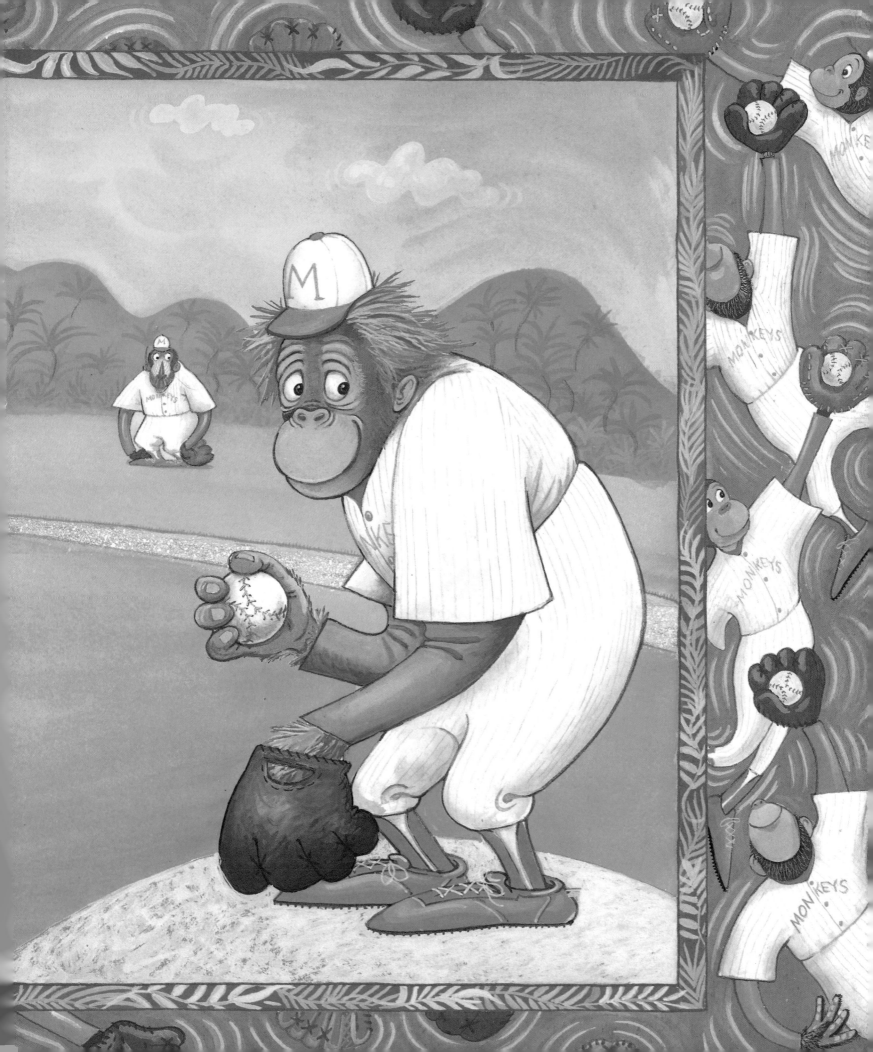

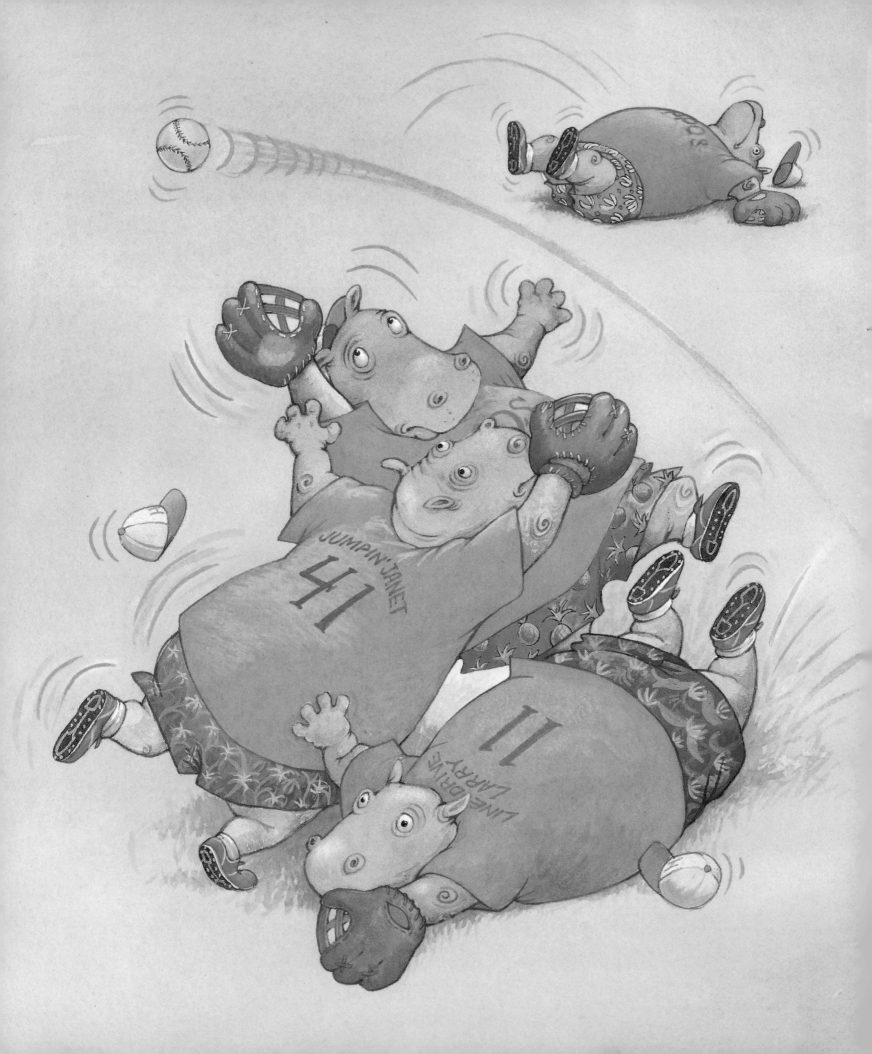

As they watched the monkeys play,
The challengers were glum.
They could *never* lick the champs;
The hippos felt so dumb.
Missing pitches, dropping fly balls,
Tripping over feet,
Nervously they thought about
The team they could not beat.

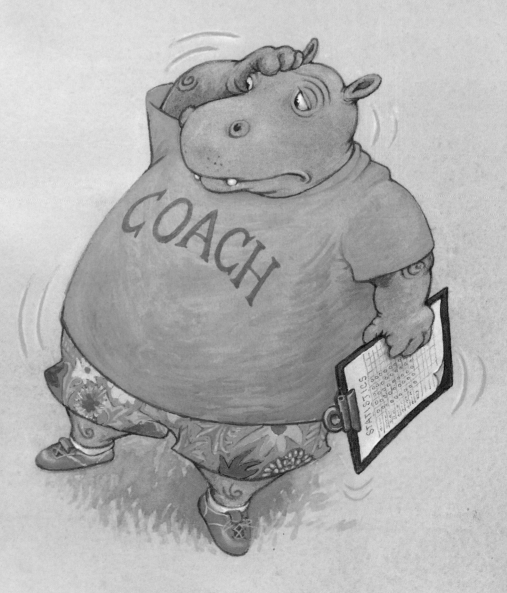

On and on the monkeys laughed,
Though no one scored a run.
Inning after inning,
They just played for fun.

Their fans were up and shouting;
Creatures whooped and cheered.
They gobbled up the hot dogs
As the popcorn disappeared.

The monkeys went on jeering
Till the hippos cried, "Enough!"
Grimly they played harder
And vowed to show their stuff.

They all buckled down and so,
In spite of their great weight,
They played so well that not one
Prancing monkey crossed the plate.

Now the hippos swung their bats
As if they meant to win,
Thundering around the bases
While their fans began to grin.

The monkeys stared in wonder.
They'd never been outdone.
Till, all at once, with four base hits,
The hippos scored a run!

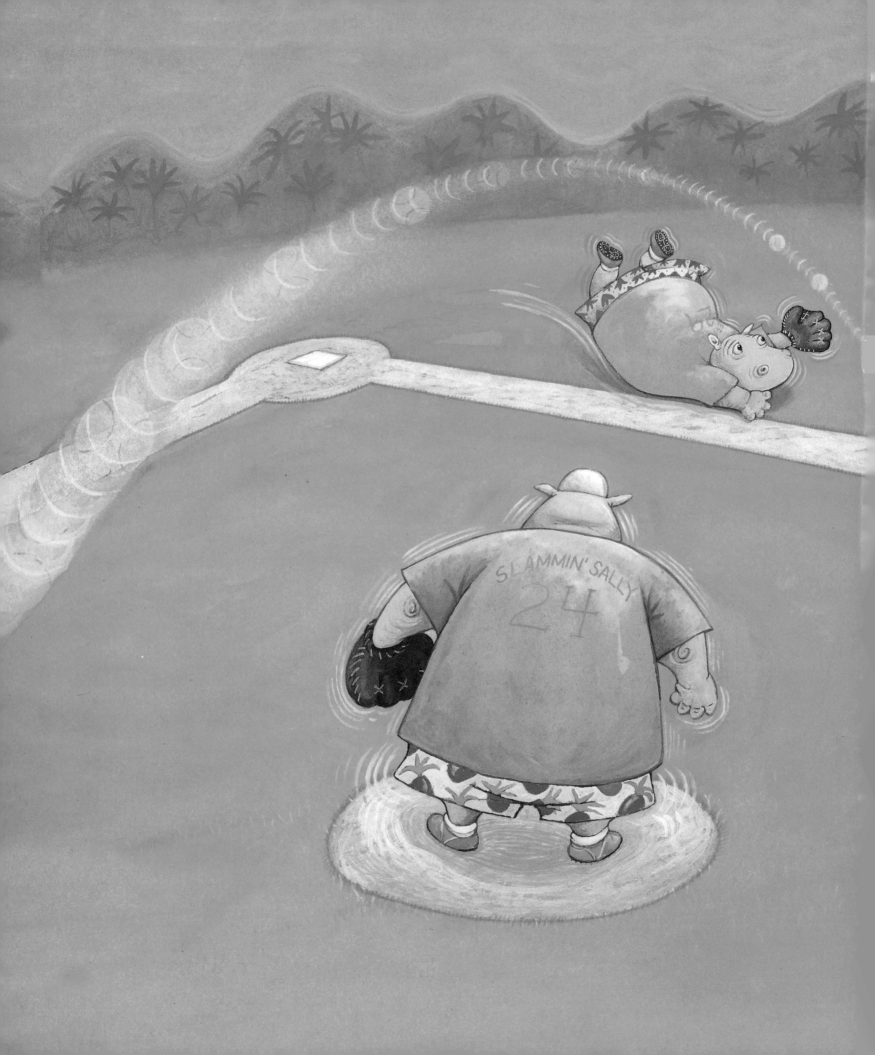

The monkeys knew they had to score
Or kiss the game good-bye.
It was now the bottom of the ninth,
Time for do or die.
First, the chimpanzee struck out;
"Strike three!" the orangutan heard.
Then a baboon got a hit
And ran all the way to third.

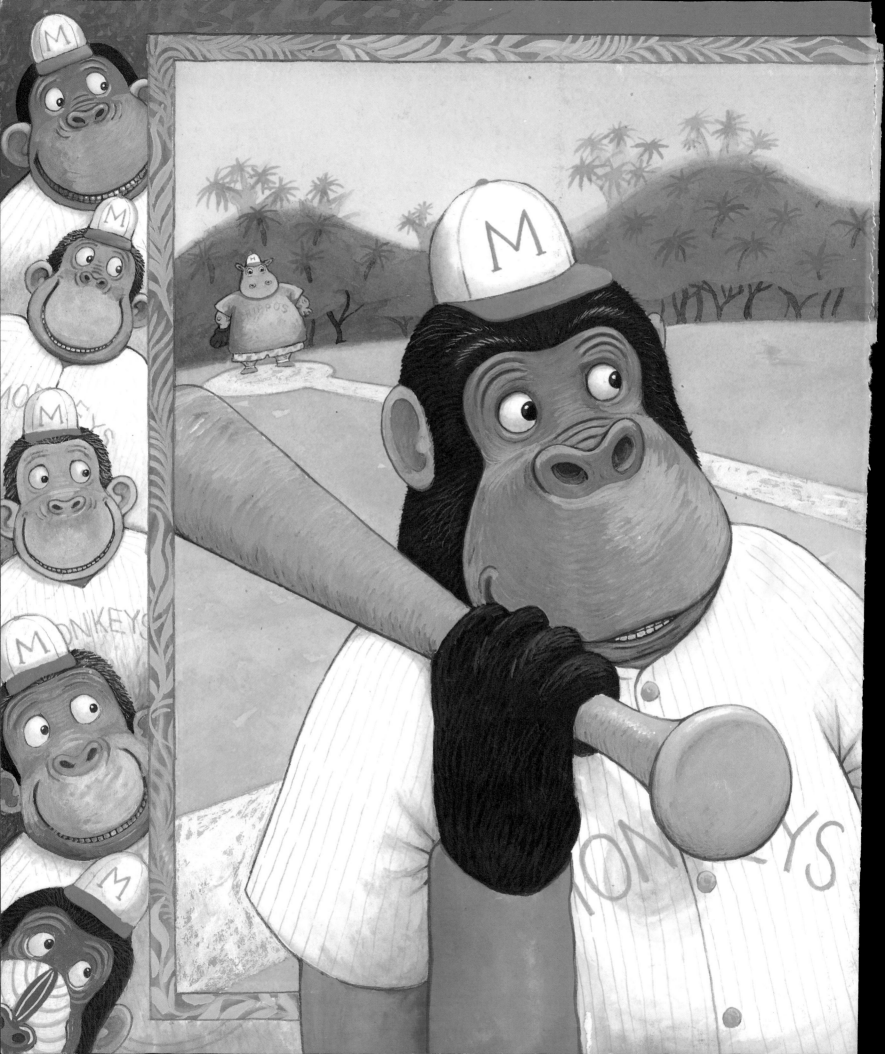

Now the monkeys saw their chance;
Their hopes began to rise.
Finally they saw the way
To beat those tubby guys.
Still, the monkeys had two outs;
Their manager chewed his hat.
He could hardly bear to look
As the gorilla came to bat.

The gorilla stepped up to the plate
And took a practice swing.
His bat looked like a tree trunk
When he twirled it like a sling.
Then the pitcher wound up,
And a perfect curve she threw.
"Strike one!" called the umpire,
And the next pitch was "Strike two!"

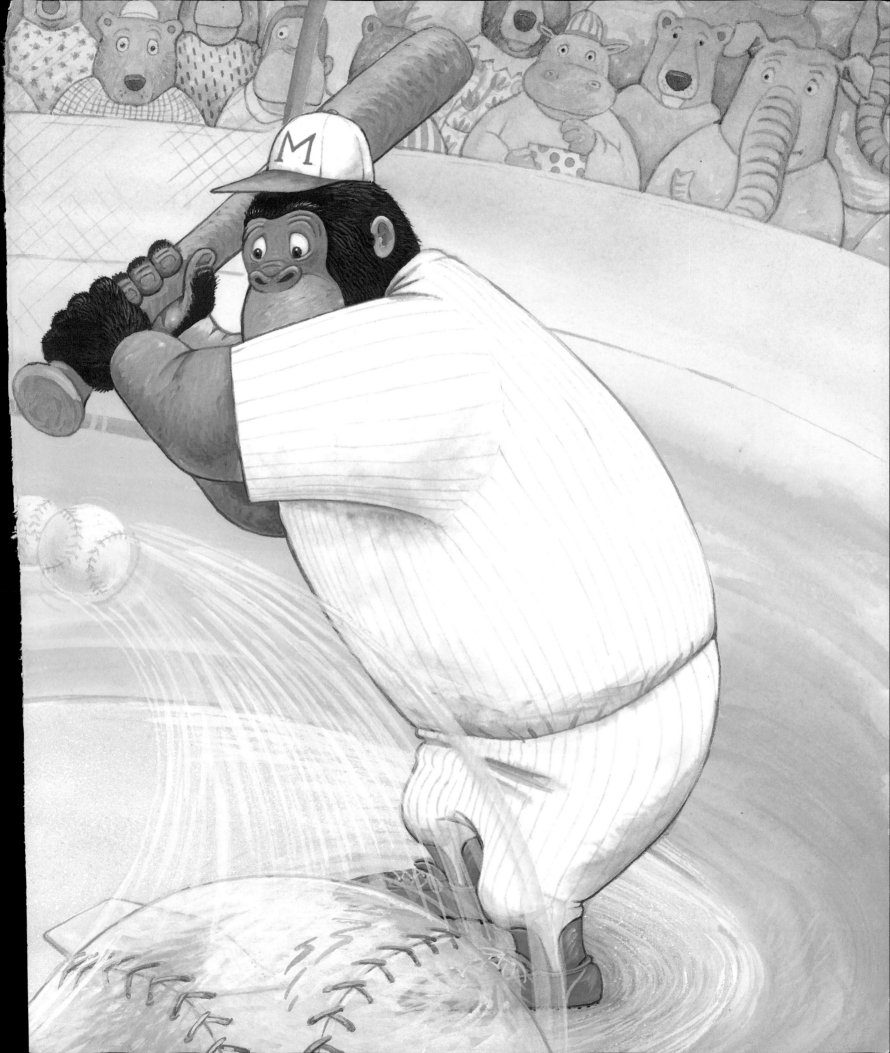

First the windup, then the pitch,
Then a splitting *crack*!
Up, up, up the baseball soared.
Would it ever be coming back?

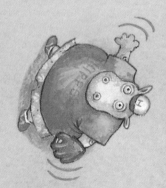

Every anxious pair of eyes
Searched the cloudless sky.
No one there had ever seen
A baseball fly so high.

When the ball headed back toward earth,
A wind came from the north.
It tossed the ball from side to side
And blew it back and forth.
Round in circles a hippo ran,
Turning and spinning about,
Until he dove and caught the ball
And the umpire yelled, "YOU'RE OUT!"

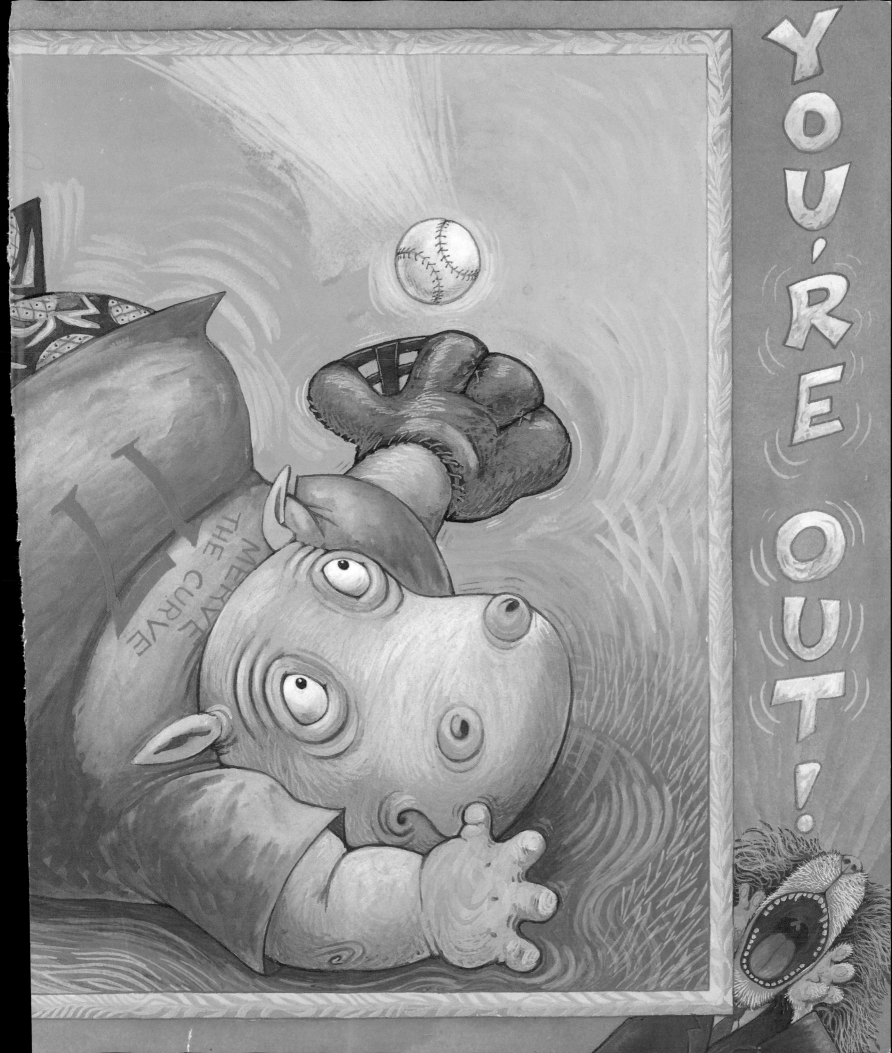

Now the game was over.
The victory was sealed.
All the jungle creatures cheered
The hippos on the field.

What a celebration
Of hippo glory, hippo fame
For the proud, triumphant winners
Of the jungle baseball game!

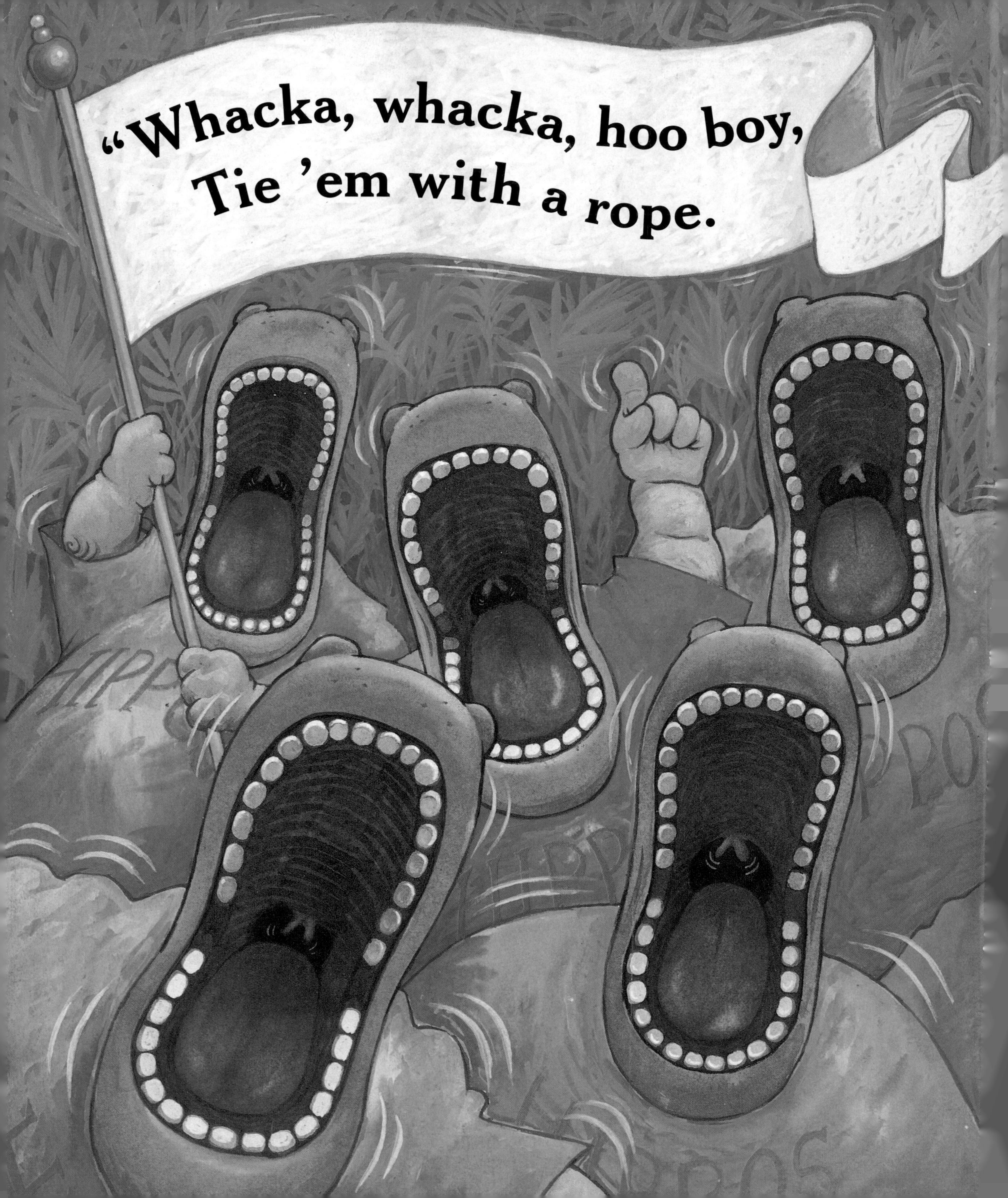
"Whacka, whacka, hoo boy,
Tie 'em with a rope.

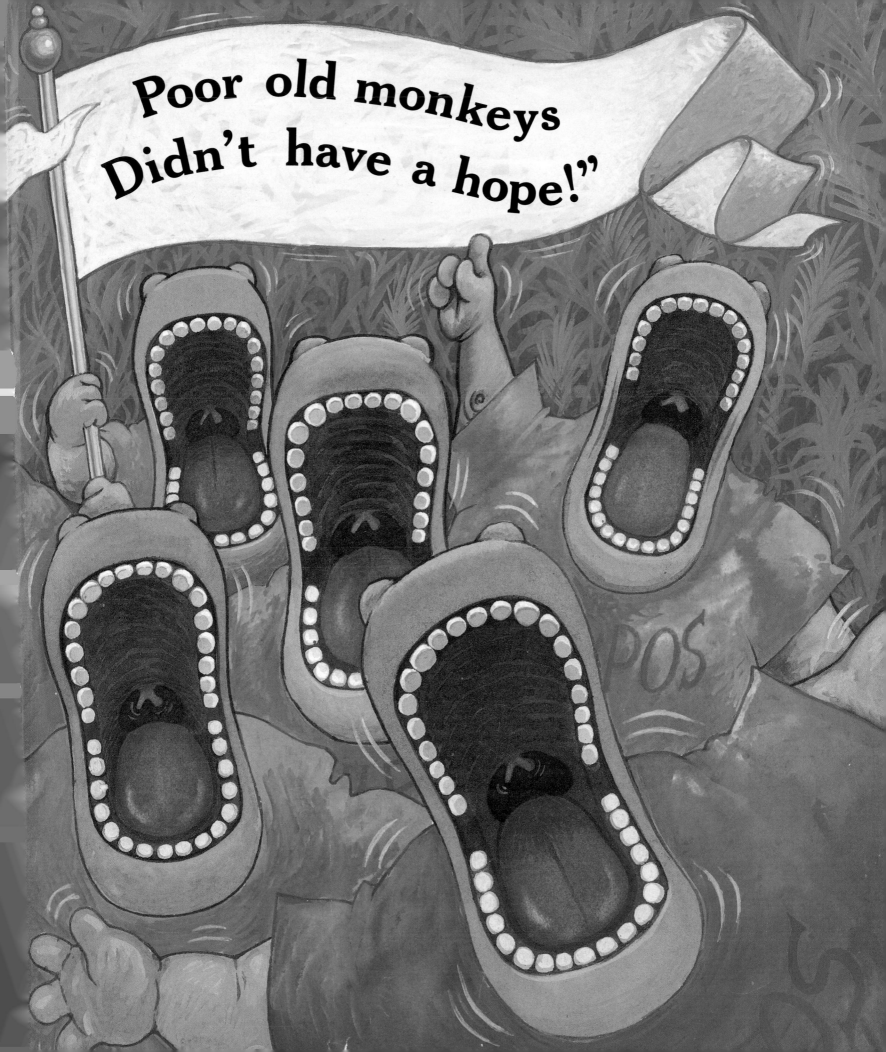

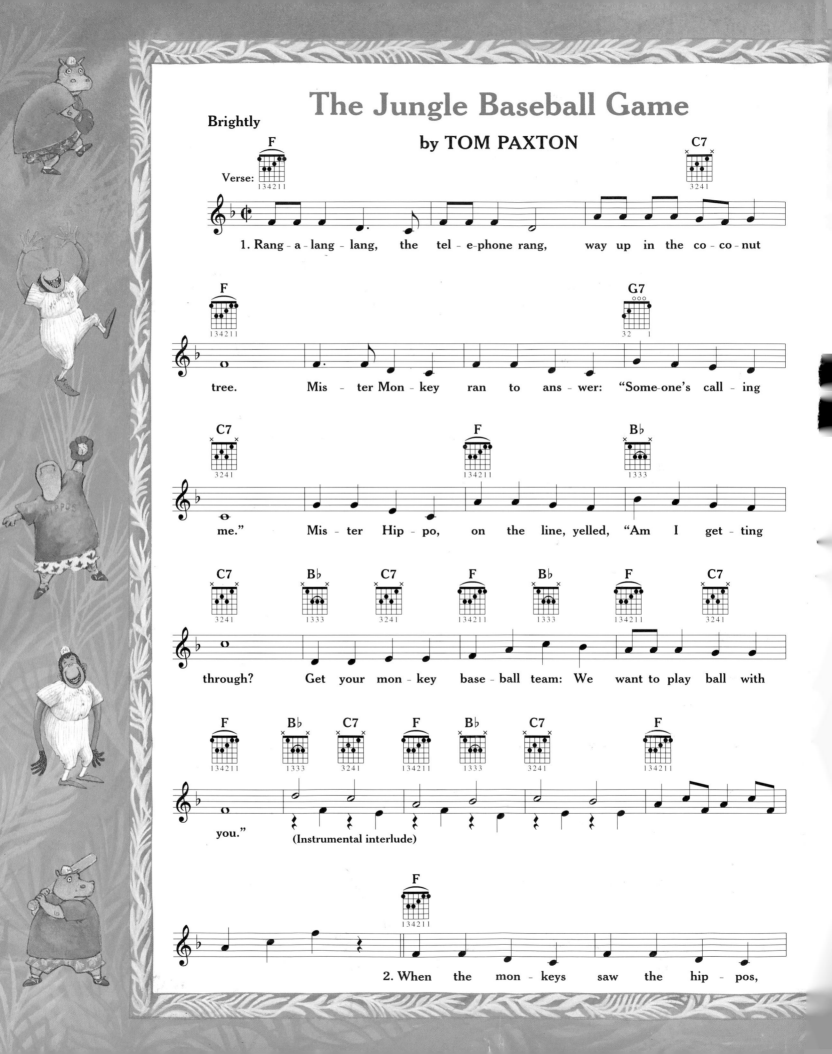